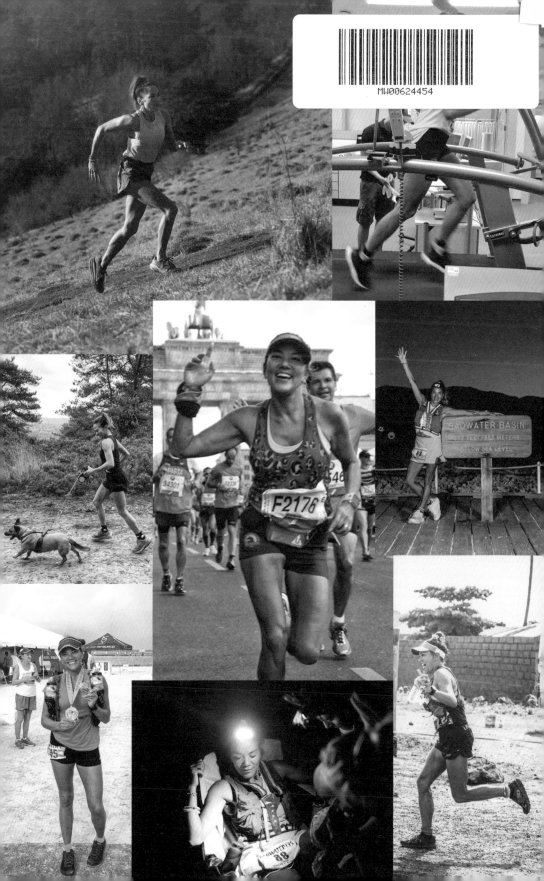

TRAILS AND TRIBULATIONS

TRAILS AND TRIBULATIONS
THE RUNNING ADVENTURES OF
SUSIE CHAN

BLOOMSBURY SPORT

LONDON · OXFORD · NEW YORK · NEW DELHI · SYDNEY

BLOOMSBURY SPORT
Bloomsbury Publishing Plc
50 Bedford Square, London, WC1B 3DP, UK
29 Earlsfort Terrace, Dublin 2, Ireland

First published in Great Britain 2024

A catalogue record for this book is available from the British Library

Library of Congress Cataloguing-in-Publication data has been applied for

ISBN: HB: 978-1-3994-0877-6; eBook: 978-1-3994-0879-0; ePdf: 978-1-3994-0880-6

2 4 6 8 10 9 7 5 3 1

Front cover image courtesy of Dominic Marley/El Carousel
Back cover images are author's own, with the exception of: Beyond the Ultimate (right)

Endpaper images are author's own, with the exception of: Left page – Haz Pics (left, second
down); Peloton Interactive, Inc./Phil Hill (top right); Beyond the Ultimate (right, second down).
Right page – Dominic Marley (top left); Peloton Interactive, Inc./Phil Hill (right, second down
and bottom middle)

Typeset in Bembo Std by Deanta Global Publishing Services, Chennai, India
Printed and bound in Great Britain by CPI Group (UK) Ltd., Croydon, CR0 4YY

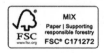

To find out more about our authors and books visit www.bloomsbury.com
and sign up for our newsletters

This book is for Lily. I love you.

CONTENTS

PROLOGUE

I am gripping the rocks for dear life.

This is unexpected. The drop to my left is deathly. I try not to look, but the part of my brain that slows to look at a car crash makes my eyes dart to my left. Past the jagged rocks below me, people look tiny on the ground. I start to feel dizzy. *Do not look!*

Instead I look at my hands gripping stone. The rocks are radiating heat into my palms, my fingernails have days' worth of dirt underneath them, my hands are dry and dusty. The desert has coated me with a thin layer of itself. I am frozen to the spot, paralysed by vertigo – and fear. One leg is tiptoed on a rock no larger than a fist. There is no place for my other foot; I swing it gingerly left to right, trying to find some purchase. Nothing. I let it hang. *Well, this is it then.* Using my fingers to grip a little harder, I pull myself forward against the tug of the heavy rucksack on my back. I'll just have to stay here until I perish.

'ALLEZ! Out the WAY!'

I genuinely cannot move. Maybe I should have paid more attention to the course. No one said anything about rock climbing. I am so tired, so very hungry. Everything aches. The sun is beating down hard on me. Breathing in to calm myself is no comfort; I breathe in just warm, dusty air.

This is not what I signed up for. My fear of heights will stop me achieving my dream. *For God's sake.* A thought flashes through my head: *What a waste of time and money.*

'ALLEZ!!! MOVE!'

I simply cannot.

1

THE START LINE

Waterloo Bridge, London 2013

'I could not walk another step.'

The rain is hitting my face as I peddle straight into it, making me feel a bit less hungover. London skies are overcast: a sea of cloud above sits oppressively on the skyline as rain pours down. Everywhere is grey.

My jeans are now fully saturated. I keep telling myself I will invest in some waterproof trousers; until then it will have to be turning up for work looking like a drowned rat once again. *How on earth am I going to get through today?* I feel exhausted before even making it to my desk. Last night I ran a half-marathon after work, swam a mile, then sank a bottle of red wine to rehydrate. Not the best preparation for the biggest race of my life, but I feel the alcohol units are offset by the amount of miles I am running. Plus old habits die hard.

The lights turn red. I squeeze my brakes and the back wheel slithers us to a halt. Rain drips down my face. Cyclists bunch up around me waiting for green. A couple ignore the lights and weave through the traffic turning on to the Strand. Another day, the same as the day before, the week before, and the month before that. Endless days like this.

It's just one month's time, I tell myself, *just four more weeks.* Will I be craving rain on my face like this?

I arrive home that day to a parcel. Something else for the race! I open it. It's a venom pump. I pop the lid of the plastic packaging open and look at the large yellow syringe with various attachable heads of different sizes. Presumably to be paired with the size of the offending venomous bite. I can't take all of those – far too much extra weight. They weigh only a few grams, but it all adds up, apparently.

'Mummy, what's for dinner?'

I'll think about venom pumps later. I rip open another 50p packet of instant pasta and sauce and put it in the pan, and flick the kettle on to boil.

'Pasta AGAIN?'

'You like pasta!'

It fills us both up and it's cheap. It will have to do.

••••

I found out about the Marathon des Sables in the pages of *Runner's World* magazine. I had been running for one year, had completed a couple of half-marathons and marathons by this point, and misguidedly considered myself something of a running aficionado.

Never seen anything like this, though: it looked other-worldly. The pages had glossy images of golden sand dunes, vivid blue skies and runners dotted like ants through the landscape. They all appeared to be wearing very similar outfits: tight silvery tops, legionnaire hats and billowing khaki things on their legs that looked like voluminous silky leg warmers. They can't possibly be leg warmers? In a desert? Trainers were not visible.

These runners were running around 160 miles in the Sahara Desert. The Sahara! It would take six days and the runners were something called 'self-sufficient'. I read the article.

'I could not walk another step,' wrote the journalist a few days in. My eyes raced through the article, taking in the details.

Each year several hundred runners head to south Morocco to embark on the race of a lifetime, a multistage race (meaning it is run across multiple days). Each day is a different distance and each day brings its own flavour of the desert. At night the runners are put up in tents to sleep, ready to do it all over again the next day.

The details made it sound even more adventurous. 'Self-sufficient' meant the runners had to carry their sleeping gear, food for the week and various items to help keep them alive in the harsh desert environments. There was no mention of a venom pump.

My interest was piqued. *Races like this exist?* I thought marathons were the longest thing a runner could attempt. Apparently not. Beyond that, beyond the famous 26.2 miles, is a whole new world – and that world is called *ultrarunning*.

Unbeknown to me looking at those shiny bright pictures of the golden desert landscape, I was about to be sucked head-first into a world that would embed itself so deeply in me. It would become part of my being and so ingrained that it would change the very course of my life, putting me on a new trajectory that I could never have predicted or dreamed of as I cycled through the rain to work.

••••

I'm pretty sure I smell like a brewery.

I tidy my hair behind my ears, pop a mint in my mouth, wander into the museum building and collect my keys from security. The same bunch every day is hanging on its hook for me. A hefty key, well over 100 years old, takes centre stage, and the rest of the bunch is like its own potted history of keys through the ages. The newest and most shiny ones are for the latest gallery where I am working. These keys unlock the doors around me.

It's 1997 and this is the place where I dreamed of working as a child: the British Museum. Millions of visitors enter through its impressive portico to be enlightened and entertained by the world-class collections from all corners of the globe. When I got the job, I could not believe my luck; it felt like winning the lottery because hundreds apply for the role of Museum Assistant. It had taken two years of working for free as a volunteer to get an interview and my starting annual wage was £10,500. That did not get you very far in central London even in 1997.

For four days a week I worked extra shifts in a local pub to get by, which had its perks: locals bought me several drinks each shift, so I could get drunk for free most nights.

And smell like a brewery the mornings after. This morning we would be moving Ming Vases off display and taking them to the cavernous storage basements which form the underbelly of the huge building in Bloomsbury. A mild hungover sweat misted my brow, but it was nothing I had not dealt with before – on most days, to be honest.

I loved this place, loved the horrendously low-paid job, loved working among the museum objects and loved my colleagues. On the evenings when I was not working in the pub, I was in a pub with them. Your early twenties are like that. It was the late 1990s and you worked hard and played hard. It felt like the whole of London was out partying every night.

The work was generally quite joyful. I love history and although I worked with the famous Egyptian mummies, walked past the history-changing Rosetta Stone daily on my way in, and handled millions of pounds worth of antiquities every single day, sometimes it was the most humdrum object that would tug at my thoughts and make me grateful for my job. A comb from ancient Sudan, a plain food bowl thousands of years old, a Japanese print depicting a simple street scene. These little snippets of everyday life from people who lived hundreds, even thousands of years ago were right in my hands all these years later. *Who used this? Who made this?* They would never have thought that centuries on someone like me would be holding the very same item. The privilege was never lost on me.

This was the life for me, quietly working away in basements, cupboards and drawers. Organising, sorting, moving museum objects around; hanging them on walls, being creative in how we displayed them. Sometimes we were the ones to take objects to other museums around the world and I dipped my toe into another life. Travelling on flights in fancy class, staying in hotels well above any budget I could afford and seeing bustling cities via the museums. A few days out of my normal life, transported into another: New York, Tokyo, Los Angeles, Paris. Then I stepped off the flight home and, like Cinderella as the clock turned midnight, was transported immediately back to my everyday life. Waiting at the bus stop to get back to my flat and worrying about not having the money for my electricity bill.

I enjoyed my twenties, partying hard with money I did not have, and enjoying my job. I worked with interesting things and with interesting people. I have always felt like the least academic person, the thickest person in the room – and generally speaking, in the circles where I worked, I was. It never bothered me, though, learning more about history by asking questions, and getting to be handy with workshop tools by building and making things for various exhibitions.

Occasionally my electricity did run out and I sat there in the dark with no money to put in the meter, but I could drive a forklift truck and build a scaffold tower, and I wasn't fazed about hanging a huge picture on a wall or moving a statue.

Things gradually changed as I got nearer my thirties. The shift was so slight, so incrementally small week on week, that it was not obvious to me.

The Saturday and Friday night parties turned into Thursdays, Wednesdays, Sundays, then daily. A bottle of wine turned into a bottle of vodka. I smoked nights away or stayed awake for 48 hours at a time, making the most of the weekends. I thought I was having fun, but actually, on reflection, it was not fun at all. I could be loud and obnoxious at times, the noisiest person in the pub. I was chucked out of some, too drunk, too loud, too unladylike. As this gradual change slowly seeped its way into my routine, I became only functional in my job. Just getting to lunchtime, then getting to 5 p.m. As long as I turned up to work on time and got the job done, no one would notice, would they?

••••

When I was 26, I became pregnant, and Lily came into my life nine months later. I can remember deliberately waiting until after New Year's Day to do the pregnancy test, an instinct deep inside telling me I was pregnant even as I wanted to go out and party the New Year in guilt-free.

A couple of days later, looking at the two lines on the test kit, I realised shit had just got real.

The morning after I gave birth, the sunrise was shining bright and cheery through the big windows of the Royal Free Hospital. We were a few floors up, and I looked over at my tiny baby, all pink and curled up, tiny hands in tiny fists, with the smallest, cutest nose I had ever seen on a human being. My heart filled with love. I picked her up and waddled over to the window to show her the world outside.

'Look! Welcome!'

I tried, I *really* tried to be a good parent. There is so much people do not tell you about being a mum. Back then, social media did not exist like it does today. Facebook was three years away from being a thing and Instagram another eight. There were no spaces to connect with people in the same position as you. Nowhere to be anonymous and talk with other people going through the same thing. Nowhere to go online and look up how you should be feeling once you have given birth. It was simply not the thing to say how hard being a mother actually was. I struggled in silence, struggled with the care, struggled with the tiredness, struggled with the bills, struggled with just how terrible I was at being a mother. Around me I saw beaming mothers rolling their luxury buggies around and relaxed couples fussing over their happy babies. I wanted that, wanted to feel relaxed, in control, confident.

Fortunately, my daughter was a good baby. A lovely child, easy, beautiful, docile yet curious in the right amounts. *Is it just me, then? Why am I so bad at this?*

The evening glass of wine reverted back to vodka. The odd roll-up out the back door escalated until life got sticky for me again. There was a moment, a really low moment, when I woke up hungover once again, fuzzy-headed and nauseous, and realised that continuing in this low-paid job, sinking wine in the evenings, getting off my face in my own company, and repeatedly trying and failing to be a better parent – things could not continue like this.

Things felt like they were hanging by a thread for me. I was deeply unhappy. *Fine, I can deal with deeply unhappy when it's just me, but it's not just me any more. I simply have to do better for my daughter.*

Within 48 hours I had walked out of the door, put my flat up for sale and started looking for a new job. I needed to be away from the bright lights and temptations of London. I so desperately wanted to be one of those confident mothers, with their fancy buggies and nice clothes. I wanted to be a better role model for my child and, most pressingly, enable her to have a better life.

I turned up on my sister's doorstep in Surrey with a few bags.

Time for the next chapter of my life. Lily and me.

It did not take me long to realise that there was no work for me in Surrey that suited my past experience. The large museums and galleries were all in London and as a single parent I could not afford the commute – the ticket or the time. I found a job in the local borough council offices. It could not have been further from my previous job: answering the phone and logging complaints from disgruntled people moaning about their neighbour's leylandii growing too tall, and fuming about the ice cream van coming round daily 'disturbing the peace'.

I hated it.

The work sucked, but my boss was funny, kind and lovely, and it covered the bills – just. I found my daughter a good school by going to church a lot. Life was dull, but dull was what I was after. Things settled down and I met a guy who also worked in the local council: he was good with Lily, got her packed lunch ready for school, pushed her swing, cleaned the school shoes. He seemed to be better at all those things than me, so when he asked me to marry him, I said yes.

I do not recommend walking down the aisle smiling and nodding at the gathered crowd, pretending this is the single happiest moment of your life while knowing in your gut that it is not really what you want.

How many people do this? I wondered, yet at that time in my life it seemed the sensible thing to do. Lily needed a bit of steadiness and this was it: a vast improvement on the last few years. It was time to play happy families.

A bonus of being married meant I could go back to working in London in the sector I knew and enjoyed. Money was not so tight and I would not be the only one if the school called for a sick day pickup.

Life plodded on. I worked for the Arts Council Collection and then moved to University College London, looking after their collections and exhibitions. There were the usual ups and downs that occur in any job, but generally I enjoyed my work and my colleagues.

Then one day, in the course of a few hours, everything suddenly and shockingly changed. My steady and boring life was thrown off the rails once again and once again I found myself trying to get out of a hole.

••••

My card was declined. Having a card declined had been a peril of the last 15 years of my life. Embarrassingly I have had it declined for less than a fiver on countless occasions, but this was my credit card, which I barely used because I was trying very hard to pay off my large overdraft accumulated in my London years and to live within my means. I asked the person in the shop to run it through again and once again it declined the payment.

Odd, but I assumed there was an error at the shop's end or a security query that was stopping payment. I made a red-faced apology and stepped outside, thinking I would phone the bank to double-check, smooth out any security questions and go back in and pay.

'The card is at its maximum.'

'I'm sorry, what?'

'You've reached your limit.'

'I don't use this card. Can you double-check?'

'Sorry, I *am* looking at the account, you are maxed out.'

With a sinking feeling, I immediately reported it as fraud. What money had come out? Where? I demanded to know how thousands can just have been spent without so much as a PIN being used.

'A PIN was used. There are many withdrawals, over several weeks, for £200.'

'Where? Where are the withdrawals?'

'At cashpoints in Farnham. Where you live.'

'WHAT?'

The card was always in my purse. This simply did not make sense.

They could not really do much, because it was over such a prolonged period of time, months of withdrawals at times when I was at home.

They flagged the account and froze the card, but told me I was liable for the money until fraud could be determined.

That evening, my husband came home and I told him about the card. He agreed it was very odd and surely the bank would be able to help me, because I had not taken the money. It must have been stolen. I was sick with worry.

The next day, I went to work as normal and from there I called my sister. She told me to look at a statement to see if there was a pattern, information on which cashpoints had been used. I did and all the withdrawals were in the evening and within a two-mile radius of my home.

I cannot believe it was the credit card people who were the ones to nudge the thought into my head. And it started as more of a question than a conclusive thought. But that evening I came home and straight out asked him: 'Is this you?'

'Don't be ridiculous! Why would I do that?'

He was convincing and it did seem unreal. *He is not that sort of person, is he? He is too quiet and unassuming. Impossible!*

Yet it was the most obvious explanation.

The seed of doubt had been sown and I asked again. How can money be spent from a card that is at my home? He point-blank refused any knowledge. Someone might have cloned my card. The card company simply had to do better.

My sister smelled a rat and asked a question: If he had maxed out my credit card and refused to admit it, where did that leave me?

I asked the credit card company. They informed me that even if he did admit it, we were married, so they were not liable for the money at all. It was between him and me, unless I could prove a crime had been committed.

I suddenly began looking at him through new eyes, questioning other details of our life. With him still denying any knowledge and looking and acting perfectly normal, I decided to call up the bank and asked for a statement on the joint account.

That too was maxed out to the limit and in debt by thousands of pounds.

These details turned out to be tip of the iceberg. It's hard to remember the order of things. He was calmly and quietly refusing to admit anything.

I felt helpless and confused. I went into my branch of Lloyds to talk to them. 'I think my husband is stealing my money. I don't know what to do.'

After a hushed conversation through the teller's window where I did my best to summarise what had just happened, I was ushered into a room. A lovely lady was saying soothing things to me as she opened my accounts and then froze all of them.

'We will see what we can do, Ms Chan. This is a very unusual situation.'

'What about my house? He's on the mortgage.'

I had purchased my house with a deposit from my dad and, despite being so skint, had never ever missed a single mortgage payment. Never. It was my house, for my daughter and me, and I had scrimped and saved to keep us there. It was not a brilliant property, an end-of-terrace, ex-council house with zero kerb appeal, but it was in a nice town and had a garden that caught the sun, and it was ours, Lily's and mine. Our home, our place of safety, the place where she would grow up.

When we married, my dad had gifted him a small share in the property.

The kind lady from Lloyds pulled up the mortgage account on to her computer. I will never forget this moment: she went white as a sheet and blinked at the screen.

'What is it? What is it?'

She did not say a word. I could see her trying to compose herself to form a sentence together.

By this point, I was in a full-on panic. I could feel the blood draining from me as I sat slumped in the chair in the little windowless office.

'Excuse me, I'll be back.'

And with that short sentence she left me alone in the room.

I started sobbing. I sat there crying with my brain spinning for what felt like an age. Just crying with frustration and helplessness. *What is happening? Why is this happening to me?* I did not understand. I felt so overwhelmed and out of my depth.

After a while she reappeared and introduced a very concerned-looking man. He was the branch manager. 'Ms Chan, I'm so sorry. I don't know how to tell you this, I really don't . . . but there are a lot of second charges against your property.'

'What? What does that mean?!'

I had no idea what they were saying by now. Everything blurred. They both looked shocked and I was crying hysterically by this point, just single words coming out in between the sobs, tears streaming down my face. They were doing their very best to make me feel better.

I have no idea how long I was in that office in Lloyds Bank, Oxford Street, but I will never, ever forget the kindness of those two staff members.

A cup of sugary tea appeared. The kind lady hugged me. The branch manager was kneeling down to my level, talking gently to me, doing his best to try to reassure me.

'Things will get sorted out. We will do what we can to help.'

The bottom line was that a load of loan companies now owned and had rights to my property, because several loans had been racked up against the address. The credit card bill was small in comparison and by now it was tens of thousands.

It must have been awful for them at the bank, but they treated me like a friend, not a customer that day. Eventually, when I finally managed to regain some dignity and stop crying, they told me to come back in tomorrow or the day after, whenever I was ready, to see how they could help, if at all. They needed to see legally what they could do and I needed to go home to collect my daughter from school.

I walked out of the branch in a daze. Fuzzy-headed from the tears and with tense knots of fear and anxiety.

By the time I stepped off the train home after the one-hour commute, I was raging. *Fuck me over, I can handle that, but don't you dare do that to my child. This is her home.*

When he walked in the door, I told him to get the fuck out. He simply turned around and shut the door behind him. I opened a bottle of vodka and a packet of cigarettes.

••••

Three days later my brother was knocking on my front door. I had not yet told him the story as the shame of the whole situation was bearing down on me. I simply could not bear to speak about it unless I had to. Just uttering one word would break me down again.

I opened the door. 'Don't you dare bale on me!'

He stepped in.

We were supposed to be running a half-marathon. A whole half-marathon. My first ever running race. Not a 5K or a 10K, but straight into a half-marathon. When I agreed, I did not even know how far it was, and when I found out −13 miles − that in turn did not really mean anything other than a very long way.

No chance. I had barely slept, had drunk enough alcohol units to sink a ship and, more importantly, did not want to run, thanks.

'Let's go, we are going to be late!'

My brother was training for his first marathon, something he had wanted to do to tick off his bucket list. He had been training well and found a half-marathon local to me, Farnham Half, and pretty much cajoled me into running with him: 'It will be good for you! Fun! You can do it.'

I had agreed without even really knowing anything about running, but why not? If he could do it, so could I!

In the past I had been on the odd run here and there; it was born out of guilt, trying to offset the bottles of wine. I vividly remember my first ever run, which I did during my lunch break at work. I left my desk, put on some gym shoes and headed out to a local park. Exhausted by the time I got there, I had paced my run by having to stop several times along the way, crossing roads and waiting for lights to change. When I arrived in the park, I decided to try to run non-stop around the two football pitches; they were big, but I thought it would be possible. Running up one long side with full gusto, I was out of breath by the halfway line and by the top corner it felt as if my heart was beating in my throat. *Sheesh, running is difficult.* I covered only a few more metres before I had to stop and hold on to my knees, bent over and attempting to regain my breath. *Is this what a heart attack feels like?* After a while my body felt calmer and I continued. It really did not get any easier, but I finally completed the full loop after one more stop to catch my breath. I walked back to the office.

Every so often I did the same run in my lunch break and after a while it was pleasantly gratifying to be able to run without stopping so much. Yes, sure it would be better if I gave up smoking, but I was not running that much and I enjoyed smoking much more than running. However, once I entered the half-marathon, I decided I'd better take a little bit more of a methodical approach to running. Perhaps try to do it more and with more consistency rather than going out once every while when I felt, momentarily, like being healthy.

Twice a week I headed out to run, not really knowing how far or how fast. I took the same route each time: out of the house and past town towards the big Tesco. The route had a few hills, and each time the aim was to run further, adding another 10 minutes.

Sometimes it was just as difficult as the previous week, but sometimes I could feel myself getting stronger, and every time I enjoyed the sensation of having completed a run. After a few weeks of this I could run without stopping for more than an hour!

Some days it was hard; being a mum meant time and enthusiasm would just disappear. The discipline wavered and sometimes the idea of running after a full day's work was not at all alluring – and if it was raining? *Forget it.*

And now, with all the life-consuming turmoil of the previous two days, I had completely forgotten about the half-marathon.

My brother convinced me to come along: 'What else are you doing?'

I looked back into my house. Lily was away with her dad. Nothing.

Within half an hour we were standing in a field on the south side of Farnham, collecting a bib number from a friendly man from the local Rotary Club. Suddenly I was extremely nervous. *What the hell am I doing here?*

A half-marathon? Now? Today? Right now?

Everyone looked like they knew what they were doing and they looked relaxed. Some had belts with little pouches of what looked like energy drinks, some carried water bottles, others were applying Deep Heat to legs and limbering up. Others had a very casual demeanour, just standing around and chatting. I looked down at my feet. I had not had the opportunity, money or common sense to buy actual running shoes. These were the same ones I wore for anything vaguely sporting, white and clumpy. I was wearing an underwired bra because the cheap Nike one, purchased in a sale, had turned out not to be at all supportive and more for show. I wore the Nike one over the top of the underwired one, as I did not want people to spot my inexperience. My outfit was finished with a tennis skirt and cheap top from H&M — both sale purchases — and I thought it looked quite natty at the time, but the ensemble felt very conspicuous in this crowd. They all seemed to be wearing thin fabric vests and shorts, and instinctively knew what to do with themselves in these minutes before the race. Many had race tops with names on them like 'Blackwater Valley' and 'Farnham Runners'.

I did not have a drinks bottle and could not recall the last time I had even drunk some plain old water. Days ago.

My brother had Sellotaped his number to his top. We both stood in the field, taking it all in.

Perhaps sensing my unease, someone came over to me and said in a jolly voice, 'I hope you like trail running!'

That was the first time in my life I had heard the phrase *trail running*.

'What's trail running?'

He laughed. 'Hills, mud, stiles — this race has it all!'

Oh, Jesus Christ.

'Just take it easy at the start! You'll be OK,' he tried to reassure me.

I'm too hungover for this.

I contemplated baling right there and then, just getting back in my brother's car and waiting for him with my eyes shut, blocking it all out, everything. Could this week get any more shit? People were gathering at one end of the field and I could sense the atmosphere had gone up a notch.

'Come on!' My brother encouraged me to the start and, before there was time for any more doubt or fear, we had started running.

••••

We were in a field running straight towards what appeared to be a solid hedge. This was not what I expected at all. Within minutes there was a slight grassy hill. My brother and I had set off towards the back of the pack and, even so, people started passing us up the hill. We did not stop to walk, though; instead we focused on running steadily rather than racing. We had both agreed not to push too hard at the start. Immediately I broke out into a vodka sweat. Next we were in what felt like forest: tall pine trees reached up skywards, forming a canopy above us blocking out a fair amount of sunlight. I noticed scents that were musty and fresh at the same time. The floor was littered with small, spiky, pine cones. The tree trunks had roots like knuckles reaching out wide, poking out of the sandy forest floor. Trying not to trip up became my next focus as I did my best to navigate my way through the woods at a run. It became engrossing, just staring at my feet, picking them up and over roots, deciding where to place them, looking at the feet and ankles of my brother in front of me doing the same.

We kept a steady rhythm for a while and then suddenly it felt like someone had opened the curtains on to a bright day. We were now somewhere totally different, a wide open field, rows and rows of crops growing in hundreds of neat, tidy lines down and away from our narrow, puddled path. Beyond the field stretched more fields, which in turn stretched into hills into the distance. We could see for what looked like miles. The ground was now more stable underfoot, so I took in the view as I ran. I was only minutes from my own house and had no idea these views and paths existed.

It continued like this for some time, the terrain varied and interesting. Sandy stony climbs where I had to watch my step, heathland with purple heather decorating either side of our route, more woods and fields. Sometimes runners ahead bunched up and stopped. *What could this be?* Stiles dividing up the path and taking us over fences. People queued and then clambered over the wooden steps to start running again straight away on the other side. This did not happen on my route to the big Tesco.

Occasionally we came out of the countryside and on to a road. In contrast to the soft trails, the familiar tarmac felt hard and solid underneath my feet. Here, spectators were gathered, clapping and cheering. Some waved home-made banners, looking for partners, family, friends. I forgot about my hangover and focused on two simple things: not stopping and not falling over.

The next thing I knew I had passed a yellow sign that read 'Mile 9'.

Mile nine!! No way?!?

This was further than I had ever run in my entire life, and right now, unbelievably, I was still enjoying it. My legs were aching like hell, the muscles felt fatigued, I had lower backache, and the sweat in my eyes was stinging, but hell, I was still running!

Spurred by the sudden realisation that I could actually do this, I could actually finish a whole half-marathon, I pushed on.

My spirits lifted, knowing that all I needed to do was put one foot in front of the other, over and over. It really was that simple: one foot in front of the other and I would finish.

The very thought of reaching the finish line gave me a mysterious new energy that I felt in my stomach and chest, and made my legs feel a little lighter again. I smiled and waved at a group of people clapping. 'Great running!' one yelled.

Me? They're clapping me?

More sandy paths, trees, hills and stiles. I had no idea where I was at all, but after a while it felt like the finish line was close. I was back on a road again and runners with medals around their necks were walking away from the direction I was headed in. Some cheered, some yelled words of encouragement. The narrow country lane was lined with a small clapping crowd. Everyone was just so happy.

Then I could see it, the finish line. With every fibre of my being, I pushed forward into the fastest run I could muster and with a triumphant smile crossed the finish line.

I had never ever in my life felt as accomplished as I did in that moment.

It seemed unbelievable that I could run that far. Thirteen miles! A medal was placed around my neck. I was utterly elated. My legs hurt like hell, but I had done it, a whole half-marathon. This was a happiness that was so pure, so proud – and all of it was mine.

My brother and I went to the pub for a lunch to celebrate. As I waited for my fish and chips, it dawned on me that I had not thought about money or debt or wanted to cry out of sadness ever since he had shown up that morning.

The next day I brought my medal into work and showed it to anyone who asked how my weekend was. Even the ones who were only asking to be polite and were not actually interested in how my weekend was.

'I ran a half-marathon!'

I had to hold on to lamp posts to step down kerbs, take the lift down single flights of stairs for days after, but I had run a half-marathon. I was a runner.

For nights after as I lay down to try to get to sleep through the anxiety of losing my home to debt collectors, I thought about that race and how running let me forget about my life, forget who I was as I focused on trying not to fall over, forget about my worries as I took in the views. I thought about how a race made life as simple as running along just trying to get to the next mile. I thought about how free it made me feel, about how it made me feel proud of what I had done, not ashamed of being hungover again. I thought about how it had brought me joy.

I looked for another race to enter.

••••

My husband admitted everything, and it turned into a confession, which I had absolutely no interest in hearing. My anger was only ever just a tiny scratch away from the surface at any given time. He was a gambling addict. Thousands and thousands frittered away on horses, football matches, fruit machines, etc. I did not care about any of it.

I cannot imagine anything so frivolous as putting hundreds of pounds on a horse race, only to lose it in minutes, and repeating the same thing over and over again in a day. But this is what addicts do and, not without my own vices, I was able to admit that a tiny part of me understood – but it was only a really tiny part of me. The second charges, the overdrafts, the credit card were just some of what had gone on. I felt sick. I would go over things in my mind: *Was that part of it? What about that? Was that real?* It was hard to know what was fact and what was bullshit. All I had to go on were my own facts, and they were cold and hard and looked like huge debt.

I struggled with telling people; it was just too painful and difficult, and no one really wanted to talk about it. Only our families knew and a couple more people that I had to let know because I was emotionally all over the place.

Could I not give him a second chance? some people asked. Not my sister or mum, who thought he was a useless piece of shit – and I agreed with them, frankly.

He sought help with his gambling addiction. His behaviour seemed to improve but I struggled hard, very hard, to find even a tiny shred of empathy or sympathy. All I had was pure anger. A burning anger and shame.

He admitted that he had intercepted my bills, torn them up and disposed of them so I could not see the increasing digits. My credit card PIN had been spied on over my shoulder, noted, and in the evenings he would wait until I was busy and take the card out of my purse, go to the cashpoint and take out the highest amount possible, and then replace the card when I was not looking.

'How did you not notice? Couldn't you tell?'

No, no, I had no clue. Yes, it was a stupid mess; and yes, it was shocking; and yes, poor everyone.

The only way I could write off some of the debt was to report him for theft. In a fit of rage one day I went to the police station, wrote down my statement on a form, and handed it to the policemen behind the counter. He read it, only his eyes moving, following the sentences of my sorry tale left to right. He looked up at me over his reading glasses with a look that was not sympathy, not unsupportive either, but more the resigned look of someone who has seen it all. I simply said nothing and held his gaze.

'I will file this.'

'Thank you.'

A pause. 'Would you like us to arrest him? We can question him for sure, but if you have proof we can arrest him.'

Yes, I would like nothing more than for you to walk into his work, or to his brother's house where he is staying, arrest him in front of loads of other people, drag him out into the street and into the car, sirens on, cuffs on, the whole shebang like on TV. Make him feel like the asshole he is, humiliate him. I want that. 'No.'

The credit card company refused to write off the debt. Everyone did. Unless I prosecuted him, as far as it looked like under law, we could have been in on it all together. I was financially screwed.

After some conversations in which I had to swallow the constant fury boiling underneath my skin, I accepted his many apologies. There were vows of paying everything back, of getting help, of it never happening again, of lessons learned.

The truth was, he was not really a bad person; he was still young and did not deserve to be hit by a maelstrom of shit even though he created all of it. He would lose his job, have nothing, and then how could he possibly pay me back?

He moved back in. Even now this is a huge regret of mine, but at the time I felt helpless and like there was no other choice. I did not have the courage or strength to proceed with trying to prosecute him, and proving it would be difficult. I felt guilty for once again disrupting my daughter's life, having spent several years trying to make it as steady as possible. I felt out of control again, and I just did not have the strength to do anything but the simplest option.

The easiest way out was to carry on and try to pay it all off. He would declare himself insolvent and all the other joint debt would be mine.

It would take years to clear, but I simply could not afford any other scenario, because I could no longer cover the housing costs solo. I hated myself for it, but back he came.

I hated the sham state of it all. I started to go out running in the evenings after Lily was in bed, and at the weekends, to be out of the house. He stayed with Lily and I ran.

Running became the thing I did for calm, to release the anger, the thing I did to feel back in control, the thing I did to stop myself getting drunk every night, because I hated being at home. I was running from the feeling that this was not the life I wanted. Running from feeling so trapped.

Running was the one thing that kept me going.

Outwardly we looked fine to everyone. All smiles at Christmas and birthdays, that sort of thing. I became a master at simply not thinking about my current situation. I became the queen of blank thoughts, occupying my mind with frivolous details. I read books that took me to different places in my imagination, and spent hours daydreaming, pretending I was living a different life, and evenings watching endless TV.

I ignored the obvious, about how I was stuck in this pointless marriage. Never thinking about the rest of the year, or the one after that. If pretending everything is fine were an Olympic sport, I would be elite. Swallowing annoyance in mundane situations became another skill, inhaling and exhaling in long, even breaths, settling my eyes on something in the distance and emptying my mind so I did not lose it. Sitting round dinner tables; chatting to school mums; small talk to colleagues – yes, the family are fine.

Then, one day I picked up *Runner's World*, and saw it: the Marathon des Sables. And I could not stop thinking about it.

I went to the bank to ask if they would lend me the money. We were on first name terms by this point. The branch manager would phone to check in on me occasionally in those early days, make sure I was OK.

'We have never had a scenario like that,' he told me afterwards. I wondered if I had become a case study.

I will forever be loyal to that bank for how they handled it, but right now I wanted to enter my first ultramarathon.

'Come on, another couple of grand is not exactly going to make much difference now! Let me do this one thing, let me have an adventure! Please!'

'It sounds dangerous.'

'Please!'

The bank lent me the money, but cancelled my life insurance.

'You'll have to get your own policy, ours does not cover things like this. Go on now, go and do your absurd adventure.'

And I was off. To the desert, to run the Marathon des Sables. A dream come true! It became my focus, my North Star, my positive force.

I was about to do something that brought me one step closer to changing my life.

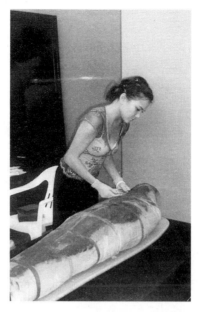

A dream come true: working in the British Museum.

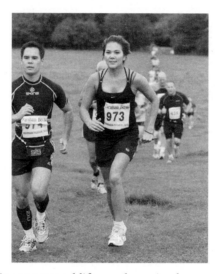

Despite upheavals in my personal life – and a raging hangover – I completed
my first ever race alongside my brother.

2

SLEEPING BAG, FOOD, WATER BOTTLES, MIRROR ... VENOM PUMP

Marathon des Sables, 2013

'Just relax and let go, Susie! Trust your feet!'

I threw myself into the training.

The Sahara Desert and the Surrey Hills are two very different places, but the hills were all I had and they were right on my doorstep. The trails became my training ground.

I purchased an Ordnance Survey map that showed trails as well as roads, and got myself a small rucksack that was vaguely designed for running (race vests as we know them were not readily available in the UK back then). Every weekend I packed some snacks and headed out. By a strange but fortunate geological coincidence, the trails around Farnham are generally sandy underfoot. Hankley Common, Frensham Ponds and the North Downs Way became very familiar to me as I ran down new and known trails, piecing together routes I had already run with new ones. They were glorious places to run, sandy in parts, muddy in others. One end of the North Downs were more closed single-track trails, with trees stooping over you and occasionally clearing to green wide fields that offered views across to the South Downs. By contrast, Hankley Common felt vast and open, and I frequently lost my bearings, adding more accidental miles to my training. Whenever I got lost, I looked for the power lines stretching overhead and then followed them, using them as a wayfinder as best I could until I hit a road.

Frensham I knew well enough and it is still one of my most favourite places to run. There are rolling sandy paths which connect and skirt around two large ponds. There are hills, evergreen trees and views across stretches of water. I loved testing myself in the white sand, pushing myself up the hills until I could barely breathe with the effort. These trails became my sanctuary.

The half-marathon had opened up a whole new world of running routes and I was eager to get out there.

I finally plucked up the courage to join a local running club. It was based in a modest, single-storey building primarily used as a local cricket team's clubhouse and sitting on the side of a small green, just south of Farnham. My first attempt at joining the club saw me make it all the way to the door, only to lose the courage to open it and walk inside. I could hear people chatting on the other side and saw more runners stepping out of their cars, coming to join the evening's run. These people had their club vests on, sky blue and maroon.

I won't be fast enough. I'll embarrass myself. I don't know anything about running. I quickly turned around and got back into my car, drove up the road and went for another solo run at my own pace – feeling rather ashamed that after getting ready and going I had not made it through the door. A few weeks later I returned, determined to make it in this time. Someone saw me lurking at the door, opened it up for me and ushered me in.

They were all very friendly and welcoming – and I did manage to keep up. It was so enabling and a revelation! New routes in every direction opened up to me. The countryside has so many places and views that are exclusively seen only by travellers on foot. This filled me with new and more exciting choices about where to take my own runs, and my running world became much bigger than just the roads. I became faster as I ran with packs of people faster than me and we went to so many races; small club races to and from the cricket club building, little local races that you entered by paying a couple of quid in cash just before they started. I experienced exhilarating and fiendishly testing cross-country running for the first time with Farnham Runners, and learned how to run downhill better just by trying to keep up with them. 'Just relax and let go, Susie! Trust your feet!'

Most importantly I made new friends, which helped me build my confidence, both in my running and in myself. Running was slowly creeping more and more into my life and taking up much more of my own time. Time that would otherwise be spent at home, drinking wine and watching uninspiring television.

••••

I entered my first ever ultramarathon in 2012. They were few and far between back then in the UK and ultrarunning itself was very much an underground sport: to get any information, you had to do a bit of digging and research. There were fewer than 20 ultramarathons in the UK, and most were a little too far for my first stab at the distance, but at least that meant there was not an overwhelming choice. Knowing a marathon distance was something I could tackle, yet being very unsure of my ability to run any further, I opted for an event that was open to both runners and walkers, and which did not operate those dreaded time cut-offs. My thought process was that I could at least run the first 26 miles, then walk the rest if necessary. It was around the coastal path of the Isle of Wight and put on by a family company called XNRG (Extreme Energy). The race itself would be across two days, and initially I wanted to do only the first of the two, but after somehow getting a friend from work to agree to take on her first ultramarathon with me, we entered to race on both days, which comprised around 67 miles circumnavigating the island. If I could not survive two days running on the Isle of Wight in June, then I would have no chance whatsoever running for six days in the Sahara Desert.

[At this point, I need to explain something: I think in miles, not kilometres. I can never figure out the conversion. So it doesn't matter what I'm running, whether the race is officially in miles or kilometres, I think in miles – and I'm mostly going to be writing in miles. Yes, I know it doesn't make sense for the Marathon des Sables, an event set up by a Frenchman and run in kilometres.]

Day 1, and my friend Emma Passmore and I ran from Cowes on the north of the Island all the way round to Ventnor on the south. It had considerably more hills than I had ever run in my entire life in one day, yet the sun shone, and with the blue sea twinkling in the sunshine next to us, the mood was jolly and positive. We made our way clockwise, ticking off 35 miles passing houses and farmland, running along beaches and along narrow paths that skirted inlets and cliffs. By the evening my legs felt utterly destroyed, tired and aching in every last part from the effort of the mileage and elevation. *How on earth will they do it all again tomorrow?*

In Ventnor we had to pitch tents to sleep. I had no clue how to do it and fumbled about trying to put poles together in a shape that resembled a tent. Emma and another runner helped me figure it out. Once done I lay down inside, trying to sleep as the wind whipped and wobbled the sides of my little camp, and my legs did their own thing – from seizing up to restless and kicking out in sudden, jerky movements.

The next morning, I woke feeling like I had been run over by a bus, and to the peculiar sound of Emma laughing manically from her tent next door.

'Are you OK?!'

'It's not normal behaviour! This is not normal!' I could hear her crying with laughter at the absurdity of what we were doing. I started laughing too. This was ridiculous! We had run over 30 miles, slept on a windy cliff slide, and were about to do it all again even though something as simple as standing up hurt. For what? A medal?

We packed up our tents and headed to the start of Day 2 to complete the full coastal path, continuing clockwise. The first few miles pained the muscles, the soreness affecting every step, but once we were a couple of miles in, the aches subdued enough for the running to flow a bit more again. The second day was supposed to be slightly shorter except we got a little lost.

Sea on the left, island on the right was our mantra, but as fatigue set in we found ourselves standing in a car park without the sea in view in any direction, so for the first time in my race running life – and definitely not the last – we had to retrace our steps and added on extra miles.

Despite the terribly achy legs, we had a blast and finished feeling elated, crossing the line hand in hand and punching the skies! We were ultrarunners!

The truth was, it was actually not that bad. Yes, you got tired; yes, your legs ached, but there were bits of walking, checkpoints laden with sandwiches and cake, views that made your heart soar, and many, many laughs along the way. I was sold.

••••

As the hundreds of miles of training ticked over, my thoughts turned towards my kit and what I needed to bring with me in the race. The rules insisted on certain pieces of kit, some of it more obvious for surviving a week in a desert – sleeping bag, food, water bottles – and some of it less obvious – a mirror, €200 in cash, the venom pump.

Every runner starts off the week with a full pack. Nutrition is crucial: a minimum of 2000 calories a day is required by race rules – if you want more, your pack will be heavier for it. As the week progresses and you get more tired, you eat your way through your pack so it gets lighter. The lighter the pack, the easier it is to run through sand.

The weight of everything you carry becomes an obsession. Each little thing adds up, so I blew my entire budget on a sleeping bag that was incredibly lightweight and packed very small. You overthink and question everything you are carrying. You weigh things obsessively.

The smaller you are, the harder it is to carry kit. Women 1.52 m tall and 51 kg have to carry the same kit as men 1.82 tall and 83 kg.

My mission became trying to find high-calorie food that weighed hardly anything and could withstand the rigours of heat and being clattered about in a bag for up to a week. I wandered down the aisles of supermarkets examining labels of random foodstuffs, pondering if they would be palatable in a desert. Macadamia nuts, I discovered, score very highly, but after testing them out on a training run, even the thought of eating them was filed under 'No'. (They're bland and somehow they dry your mouth out as you chew them. Just no.)

I found some salty pretzels which had been made even more calorific and salty by being fried and were a whopping 600 calories per 125 g bag. They seemed robust too, so in they went.

Experimenting with freeze-dried food also became a pastime, swapping packed lunches at work with pouches of camping food to test. Apparently hard cheese lasted well in the conditions of the Marathon des Sables, so I tested that out by leaving a lump of it in a bag for a few days; it still tasted good and didn't lose too much shape, so it made the cut. Fatty and salty, one lump per day would be a treat.

I dithered and changed my mind about kit. We had to be prepared for day upon day of running through the heat of the Sahara, and for the temperature to plummet at night, when it could be chilly. Research had told me a material called Tyvek was incredibly lightweight and had a warm quality to it. It is used heavily in museum work to wrap and protect objects, and I had used it all the time. Now I purchased a Tyvek onesie. When it arrived it was indeed incredibly lightweight, weighing just ounces. I put it on and glanced at my reflection in the mirror. I looked like a forensic scientist, the kind you see in police dramas. *Am I supposed to hang around the race camp like this in the evenings?* After chopping the legs and arms down, it looked slightly less silly but had lost some of its warming qualities. I could not now replace the cut legs and arms, though, and it still warmed my body, so it was packed.

I cut down an acrylic compass to as small as possible on a bandsaw at work, purchased a kid's toothbrush and also cut that down, to just the bristled top half. I decided on just the single pair of spare socks for the entire week.

The kit was slowly coming together, and then swapped, and then reconsidered, and then overthought, and then changed again. It was nearly impossible to decide on what was required without being there and doing the thing. I avoided Facebook groups where people talked about shoes being ripped to shreds by dunes and the need for sand googles against potential sandstorms and, even worse, camel spiders.

Another huge unknown was the route. The race remains roughly the same format, but the distances and route change each year. It is always in the same area of Southern Morocco, near the border with Algeria, remote and dusty. In the summer, temperatures average in the mid 40s, so this race takes place in April when the weather is typically warm to hot and the seasonal sirocco winds are likely to bring sandstorms. In April the temperature fluctuations at night mean it can get cold, something you will feel all the more with the contrast to the hot desert days and if you have been on your feet for hours trying to run a multistage race.

I'll just have to wait until I'm there to find out my running fate.

The British contingent met up for the first time in Gatwick Airport on the way out. Some people arrived in groups and knew each other; some like me had loosely met up with people making up the group for our tent, which slept up to eight. People were chatting with a mix of anticipation, bravado and excitement.

I entered this race alone, and someone reached out to me on social media to suggest I joined them and the tent he was putting together. I had just made an account on social media and had gingerly started documenting some random bits of training. His name was Mark, he seemed to have a few people together for a tent and they were relatively local. Once you have decided your tent mates, you are with them for the week. They are crucial to how much fun you have around all the running. I didn't know these people, but I didn't know anyone, so I agreed. Luckily for me I struck gold: a solid, easy-going bunch of guys who offered the perfect mix of banter and support.

From Gatwick we travelled to a town called Ouarzazate – perched right on the edge of the desert in southern Morocco, it's incredibly picturesque and used frequently for film locations. It's a reasonable-sized town filled with low sandy-coloured buildings, shuttered shops and a winding souk with brightly coloured bowls, pointed silver teapots and piles of pungent fragrant spices displayed in perfect pyramids. It already felt hot and we had not entered the desert properly yet.

I had not slept very well. Now the spare time prior to the race start gave me more time to procrastinate and ponder some last-minute changes to kit before I boarded one of a long line of coaches that were to take us into the desert proper. The coach engines rattled into life and I watched the fancy hotel we were staying in disappear from sight. As we travelled out of town the buildings become more sparse, and the landscape opened up into a rocky, dry and seemingly endless nothing.

Someone from the Marathon des Sables organisation was on board our coach. They walked down the aisle, handing out the roadbook to each of us. *This is it.* This was where we found out just what each day looked like, how to navigate through the landscape, and just how far it was to our finish line. The finish line I had now been dreaming about for months.

I opened it up.

Inside was a large geographical map for each day, accompanied by a hand-drawn map. The geographical one was useless to me, because it displayed a huge area, featuring land gradients; it might as well have shown me the moon. The hand-drawn version was the one with the detail, and drawings in a friendly cartoon fashion, which made everything look very approachable and doable.

'This will be your bible for the race,' the rep told the coach. 'This is what to use if you lose your way.'

I looked at the arrows pointing through tufty grass and ripples of sand dunes.

'You must carry it with you at all times!'

I knew for a fact I did not have the skills to navigate my way out of a desert, compass and roadbook or not. It must have weighed at least 100 grams, the same weight as a medium snack.

This year's edition of the race thankfully looked like it had no surprises and followed a well-trodden format. The first day would bring a bit of everything: light dunes, small rocky hills, long desert flats that were hard underfoot and riddled with small, sharp rocks. The second day was more technical with a high mountain climb but shorter in distance; the third day much like the first, just a little longer. Everyone flicked through those first few days, wanting to get to the one day we were all talking about. I turned the pages to Day 4.

Day 4 is the ultramarathon day. This is always the longest stage in the race and can vary in distance by up to 20 miles. It looked long, but not impossible, about 50 miles with some big dunes in the last third. At least, I thought they were big dunes; they looked bigger than others in the cartoon pictures.

This was the day where you could bring some strategy to the run, as you had until three in the afternoon the following day to finish. So, well over 24 hours, which gave the option to stop for a few hours' sleep and then continue in the morning. I had decided, like most, to finish it all in one go, meaning I could get the stage over and done with and enjoy a longer rest.

After that, there was just the marathon stage and the 'fun run' last day, which was only a few miles.

I had planned what I was eating, how I was tackling each stage, exactly what kit I would be using – this without having set foot in a desert, let alone tried running in one. The race had loomed so large on the horizon of my life, taken up all my spare time, and filled my thoughts daily. To finally be on my way to the start line seemed surreal. To finally be living it felt like a dream. This was something exotic and daring, an adventure which just did not happen to an average person like me. I tried to keep my mind busy and my demeanour engaged and light with those around me on the coach, but the truth was that I had no idea what I was doing here; the feeling of imposter syndrome was almost overwhelming.

••••

Camp, or Bivouac as it was called by the organisers, was like a small village. Having seen pictures, I knew what to expect visually, but the reality was more impressive. After several hours on the road the coach finally pulled off and drove for a short time over the hard-packed desert ground, blowing up huge plumes of dust after it. We were told to disembark and picked up our luggage. From here we were to make our way to camp and select a tent with our tent mates, then advise the race staff of our tent number and who would be dwelling in it for the week. Once the tent and tent mates were reported, we were locked in to the same tent and same people for the rest of our time in the Sahara. No changes were allowed. You have to really hope you get on and that no one has any unsavoury or annoying habits!

The tents were formed in a horseshoe shape, and there were around 150 in total, divided up by nationality. About 1300 runners, who were predominantly male, would be living in very close quarters together. The inner arc of the horseshoe was mainly French, but there were also Chinese, Australian, American and a few others gathered at one end. The outer arc, enjoying the view outwards into the desert and being the most battered by any wind that might be sweeping through camp, was made up by the Brits, the largest number of competitors.

In addition to the tents for the race participants, Camp always features an admin tent, a doctor's tent and a whole area cordoned off from those taking part – the HQ. This holds the communications area, a large dining tent for all the race staff, race staff meeting tents, and a media hub, and it was home from home for over one thousand race staff.

Staff include those who do the catering, the media crew to film and record the event (shown on French TV), two helicopter pilots, two airplane pilots for emergencies, camp security and refuse collectors ensuring no trace of the event is left in the desert. By far the main body of staff are the incredible Doc Trotters, who come in their hundreds. All qualified medical staff, these volunteers man the checkpoints, dish out water and rehydrate ill people with IV drips, but mainly fix hundreds of feet shredded by the sand. There is even a dentist. Camp is vast.

Each day this whole village is flattened down, packed away, put on transportation and moved in convoy to the finish line of the next day's stage. Here, it is set up in the exact same orientation so everyone knows where to go to their tent. This huge logistical operation is undertaken by the Berbers, local to the area, and they work extraordinarily hard for the race duration.

••••

In 2013 the way to secure a good tent was to get off the coach and run the fastest you would run all week. Naturally, some tents just sat closer to the start and finish line, and these were coveted: once the race gets going, feet are blistered and bleeding, and these tents save you valuable minutes every day when you will not be walking.

As soon as the coach pulled up and gave people their luggage, it was a free-for-all, people running fast in every direction, trying to figure out the camp orientation and bag a good tent – all while dragging or carrying their luggage. I was not prepared for this at all, hauling my wheelie luggage through the sand and just trying to work out what was going on and where everyone had gone. I finally caught up with my tent mates. We had got wind of the bunfight for a good tent and as soon as the coach pulled up sent our fastest runner, Warwick, to secure ours. None of us had ever done the race so it was hard to tell if we had secured a good spot or not, and that was not really what was on my mind, because for the first time I was looking at the tent.

Tent is really a very generous description – at least, I'd come from Farnham and it didn't occur to me that the type of tent that will work in a wet, soggy field in England isn't the kind of tent that will work in a desert. I thought I was looking at a blanket on sticks. The only place you could stand up was in the middle, where the longest stick held up the thick woven black cloth that was our covering for the week. Either side from that was tapered down to the floor and secured at both ends with long sticks simply laid down on the fabric. In the front were a couple of rudimentary guy ropes. It was completely open at both ends, offering a view out onto the desert at one side and into Camp on the other. Turns out this is a design that takes into account the high winds that can cross a desert – and it can also be easily put up and dismantled. The wind resilience would be severely tested in the coming week.

The floor had a rug on it, which was as dusty as just lying down directly on the sand, and underneath were a million small rocks, all of which could be felt through the rug. (I had been somewhat ridiculously expecting the desert to be more like a beach.)

This was our home for the week. My kind tent mates graciously let me pick where I wanted to go. I settled on a spot second from the centre pole, basing this decision entirely on an uneducated guess about the least likely place for a camel spider to dwell.

This first night is the only night when runners can benefit from their luggage. The next day is Admin Day, when we surrender our suitcases and are left with only our self-sufficient race kit for the week.

Other people had thought this detail through better: pump-up beds appeared, huge amounts of food were pulled out of suitcases, actual slippers materialised. Some people relaxed in relative luxury. I did not have extra food, but it was not all bad, because we were going to be fed in the dining tent for the next couple of nights before the race started.

The food was perfectly carb-heavy: I opted for pasta and bread and more pasta and more bread. We were allowed to have either water, beer or wine with dinner. So French. Naturally I went with wine.

On Admin Day we were all funnelled through a very organised process. At the beginning we handed in our suitcase, to be taken back to await us in the hotel after the finish. This felt momentous to me, a firm line drawn, bringing an end to any more faffing and changes to kit, any vaguely decent outfit, and my phone. The race is 'phone-free' to enable a more Camp-like feel and minimise distractions. Outside communication is very limited. There is hardly any signal in the desert anyway. Handing over my phone somehow felt very final – this was it, just me in the wilderness of the desert.

Next, all of our kit was examined to make sure we had everything required, right down to the 10 safety pins. The whole bag was weighed and noted.

Then it was on to the paperwork, where we handed in our waivers and the results of a compulsory ECG which allowed us to race. Finally, we were given our salt tablets and firm instructions to take them very regularly. The last bit was to be tagged up with lanyards on retractable elastic. These had to be handed in to each checkpoint and the hole punched to record progress. Then we were given a distress flare 'for emergencies'.

I had heard rumours about the flare being rather cumbersome – and it did not disappoint. It was like a huge stick of dynamite, and I had no idea which was the firing end and which was the end to hold, and it felt like it weighed a tonne. *Where the hell am I going to store the thing?* My rucksack was packed to the brim. Lastly, we were given our race bib and had our photos taken.

The whole process took a good while, and by the time I came out the other side, I was wearing my race kit and carrying my race bag, which now felt considerably heavier than anything I had trained in, and I was hungry and thirsty all over again.

••••

Camp settled down for the evening before the big day. We lay down, lined up next to each other like dusty sardines facing out to the desert. Jokes were cracked, conversation flowed and there was a quiet excitement buzzing around camp. This was it, the last night going to sleep on a full belly, with normal feet, feeling energised.

Sunset stretched out in the sky above us. Blues turned into oranges, pinks, reds. As the light changed, so did the view. The desert was stunning; I had not realised just how beautiful it was. I took one last look out as the sunlight finally evaporated behind the mountains and turned to sleep. *This is it, the notorious Marathon des Sables. What is about to happen? What am I about to feel, see and do?*

Only one way to find out.

The stars flickered on, one by one, until the sky was filled with thousands of twinkling lights. I pulled my bandana down over my eyes, going to sleep in the Sahara Desert. A place like no other.

Dawn, Day 1. I pulled the bandana away from my eyes, and despite having it over my entire face as I slept, my mouth, nose and eyes were crusty from the sand. My mouth was gritty. I blinked and rubbed my eyes. The view from yesterday was much the same, majestic and sweeping desert, an orange dawn rising up, throwing its golden glow across the sand – which this morning was also dotted with males urinating just a few metres away. I did not realise that there were grown men out there who still pull their shorts all the way down to their ankles to piss.

I heard a strong northern accent from the tent next door. 'Eeeeee, there's a man over there walking about just in trollies.'

I had no idea what 'trollies' meant so I looked up and saw a man wandering around wearing the tiniest pair of pants I had ever seen on a grown man. He was just sauntering around with the most majestic backdrop of a giant sand dune behind him.

Welcome to the Marathon des Sables.

••••

I tore open my breakfast, a packet of camping muesli, and once again I was one step behind those who had thought this moment through better than me. We had not even set off, yet we were self-sufficient from this daybreak onwards. Many people had packed a feast to set them up for the first stage. I saw huge vacuum-packed sandwiches, salami, a tube of Pringles. Smart people who must have overpacked for today's breakfast, knowing that once they had eaten it, they did not need to worry about running with the extra weight.

I looked down at my powdery, bone-dry muesli. All I had to put in it was water. It was about as appetising as eating the sand underneath my feet.

This was breakfast on Day 1 and it had dawned on me that my whole meal strategy was wrong, and there was absolutely nothing I could do about it now.

The time had come to make our way to the start line. The Race Director, the effervescent Patrick Bauer, was there. Standing on top of a Land Rover, microphone in hand, he was bouncing around and throwing shapes to the sounds of pop music coming out of two large speakers perched either side of the vehicle.

Occasionally he joined in, singing with a heavy French accent. His rosy cheeks were shining and he looked like the happiest man alive. This race is his baby, his brainchild. In fact, he was the pioneer: for some reason Patrick decided he wanted to cover 220 miles of the Sahara Desert, on foot, alone, and self-sufficient back in 1984. His pack weighed in at a hefty 25 kg more than mine – a total of 35 kg. He was 28 years old when he embarked on that first journey, having previously discovered the desert as a roaming encyclopaedia salesman. Ten years later there were 1500 people toeing the start line of the now notorious Marathon des Sables, claimed to be one of the toughest footraces on Earth.

He beamed down at us assembled runners, hooded in desert caps, billowing gaiters protecting our feet from the sand seeping into our trainers, weighed down by rucksacks filled to the brim.

I had decided to be a little different with my gaiters. Only a couple of firms made them out of a non-rip parachute material. These were then stitched directly on to your trainers. All the ones

I saw were a dreary sandy colour, so I called up the company to see if they had something more interesting colour-wise.

'Well, I have a pretty good material that I could make them out of in pink.'

'Any other colours?'

'That or brown.'

'Let's go pink.'

At the start line my bright pink gaiters really stood out. Several people had already commented on them just as I walked to the start line.

There was a huge air of anticipation and confidence; people were happy. Patrick went through some race instructions, detailing things to look out for on the course that day, and told us how to use a distress flare: 'Point it to the sky and release the catch!'

I didn't really fancy being so distressed that I needed to use it, and I still wasn't sure I would point the thing in the right direction and not at my feet, but it was buried in my bag by now.

I looked up at the big white arch emblazoned with the words '28th Marathon des Sables'. It looked just like I had seen in photos.

During training, I had been so anxious: *Am I running enough?* When I thought about the race, it was often: *Do I have the right kit?* Something so large had been occupying my thoughts so frequently, and now it didn't feel surreal to be there. Looking at that start line arch, looking around me at all the fellow runners, I suddenly felt that this was exactly where I was supposed to be. At this start line, thousands of miles from rainy Surrey, in the Sahara Desert.

I was surprised by this feeling, having assumed I would feel nervous. Instead, I was calm, excited about this adventure ahead. Right there and then I had found a new confidence in myself.

This is my moment.

Patrick was building up his speech. People were cheering – and then it happened. The sound of AC/DC's 'Highway to Hell' blared out the speakers and everyone starting singing along . . .

'I'm on the highway to Hell / On the highway to Hell . . .'

With poles waving in the air, bandanas twirling in hands held aloft, and hundreds of people cheering, the starting klaxon went off. With a real thrill inside of me and now bursting forth from my chest, I ran under the arch to begin the biggest race of my life.

••••

The Sahara Desert dazzled me with its beauty. It changes so much as you move through it. Expecting nothing but curving golden dunes, I saw a rich variety of landscape as the panorama shifted with the miles.

We traversed around the feet of rocky jebels (mountains). The different types of rock were fascinating. There seemed to be every type imaginable here. All different shapes: some were smooth, round boulders; some sharp and angular; some were huge and imposing but on closer inspection looked like they were made up of much smaller rocks, squeezed tight together like dry stone walls. Their colours ranged from grey to brown to gold, and these in turn changed as the sunlight shifted from soft morning to searing overhead brightness, then on to an evening glow.

There were more signs of life than I imagined too. Small patches of dry-looking trees casting very little shade, wispy grasses sprouting out of shallow dunes, thorny bushes with spikes so sharp they ripped anything they came into contact with. I marvelled at the patches of greenery somehow finding a way to grow in this arid sparseness, under a strong sun.

The sun was relentless. I finally understood what it meant to have the sun beat down. Its rays were like a sweltering cloak. The heat was oppressive, claustrophobic. By the middle of the day, you could feel heat making its prickly way up your chest into your throat. There was the occasional breeze, but that brought no refreshment, just more heat.

And then there were, of course, the dunes.

They arrived suddenly into the scenery. Hard-packed stony paths abruptly changed to sand dunes, like the land meeting the sea. You were making your way around a mountain, or running across a solid dried-out lake, the ground splintered into large cracks by the heat, when all of a sudden there they were: stretched out in front of you in all their majesty, silky sides building to a crisp point snaking its way towards the horizon. When the wind struck up, it skimmed along the top of the dunes, so on closer inspection their surfaces were not as defined as they appeared from a distance, tiny sand particles being gently roused by the air and shifting ever so slightly, skimming the surfaces. The dunes were in constant, microscopic motion, ever-changing and slowly moving across the desert, millimetre by millimetre. Creeping their way across the land, they move up to several metres in a year. This means that what you see on one day is there in that moment only, your own personal snapshot.

••••

I enjoyed the first day. The heat was tough, but both the scenery and chatting to people as we went along was keeping me occupied. I had diligently been attending hot yoga classes in the lead up, for my heat training, and it was paying off. The temperatures felt manageable. The only bit of kit I was just not getting on with were the sunglasses. I was wearing a legionnaire hat − a cap with a sort of cape coming down either side of my face, covering my cheeks and neck. It flapped around as I ran and narrowed my view, muffling my hearing. This, paired with the sunglasses and the heat which was at times stifling, left me feeling a little enclosed. The hat could not be removed, because it was protecting me, the only thing providing shade, but I wanted to be able to see the desert in its real colour, not through a grey tint.

So, I decided to remove the sunglasses for the rest of the week, opting for blinking into the blinding brightness and seeing the Sahara in all its unshielded glory − the way you do when you have no understanding of the desert and are not at all sensible, all things considered.

I was half-blind by Day 2. The first thing I did was put in my contact lenses. This was a delicate task, tricky to do cleanly as a fine film of sand covered literally everything. Fine sand was in the atmosphere, floating around in the air, clinging to anything it touched. As soon as I took the lens out of the case, it would be covered in tiny grains. I had brought lenses that lasted one month, as daily replacement lenses were quite expensive and I was ridiculously worried about the extra weight. I had not taken into consideration that there are simply no clean spaces to store contact lenses overnight (yes, I know). Each morning, I sat up in my sleeping bag and washed the grime from my hands in a minimal splash of water from my drinking bottle, then carefully balanced the tiny contact lens case on my thighs inside my sleeping bag to keep it out of the air as much as possible. The most delicate part of the procedure was to transfer each lens out of the case and into my eye as swiftly as possible, using no mirror and trying to do it without getting more than a few specks of sand on them on the way up to my eye. Every attempt since arriving in the desert had resulted in sand directly in my eyes and blurry teary vision for a short while as the grit worked its way out. There were tears every morning before I could see. On Day 2, too much sand in one contact lens meant it just ripped – and was now unusable. I put the other precious lens in one eye, and that was that for the week.

From that moment on if I wanted to see anything clearly, I had to close the one eye so I could focus through my only contact lens.

••••

Day 2, and there was a lot of chatter in Camp about the climb. At the race start line, after bouts of dad dancing and a round of 'Happy Birthday' to those celebrating, Patrick warned about 'technical challenges' and advised us to take things easy.

I opened my map book to Day 2 and looked at the route. The journey was shorter than the day before, but had what looked like a miniature mountain in the middle. I'm not good with heights, never have been. When things feel too high, my legs just turn to jelly. I had no idea there was anything like climbing up a mountain in this race. *I do not have a good feeling about this.*

Off we went again, into the sandy landscape, and after several miles I saw the runners stretching out in front of me, in pairs and single file, across an enormous salt flat – and looming ahead of that, a huge mountain. It looked massive, insurmountable. My eyes traced the single file of runners making their way directly up the beast. I gulped. *This might be my undoing.*

I followed the train of runners until I got to the foot of the mountain and started the climb. At first, it was gradual and relatively steady, a mix of sand and rock underfoot. *This seems OK.* Then it started to get steeper with less sand and larger rocks. We were gradually getting higher and I turned to see my progress, immediately regretting it. *Shit, we are quite high up.* I could feel fear rising from my stomach. I persevered, slowly, and could feel my heart rate shoot up with the anxiety and effort.

After a while there was nothing but rocks to get up and over. I looked up and saw there was still a way to go, yet the route got narrower and was in parts vertical. The climb became even more perilous, and then there was a rope tethered to the rocks and fixed all the way up to the mountain top. Runners were pulling themselves up on the rope and on to the pinnacle, one after the other. *FUCK THAT!*

I felt the blood drain from my face, dizziness and anxiety rising in its place. In a convoy of single-file runners, I tried to stay in step, and attempted to get up and over a huge rock above me. Then it happened: sheer panic.

I was gripping the rocks for dear life.

The drop to my left looked deathly. I started to feel dizzy. *Do not look!*

'ALLEZ! Out the WAY!'

My mind was racing. I could not go back down; I could not step up.

How do I move from this point? How can I?

I've failed. All that work, all that effort to last a day and a half. It cannot end like this. Please, God, no.

If I did not get to the summit, I would fail. I did not put in all that money, all that effort to fail – surely not? As I hung there frozen, contemplating how on earth I could get past this, I suddenly felt a hand under my foot and one on my bum, and then I was given a firm shove upwards. I landed chest down on the small ledge, with my feet dangling down. I shuffled myself up and sat to one side.

'See! You can do it!'

A friendly face smiled at me. 'Come on, not far, just keep looking UP!'

I struggled to stand up on very wobbly legs and reached out to the rope. This was the last section of the climb, the last 20 m. I was holding on to the rope, but it was moving and bouncing with all the tugging and pulling of those slightly further up than me and it felt horribly unstable. I clung to it with both hands; it was the only thing to grasp. As it swayed, my already white knuckles bounced off the rock, grazing them and making them bleed, but I did not let go.

HOLY SHIT.

Come on, just do it, JUST TRY.

I swallowed several times over, feeling my own panic – a large lump that just would not clear from my throat. I pulled hard upwards and my jelly legs came with me. With each effort I was getting a little closer to the top, until there were just a few more steps.

There was a race official at the top. He had spotted my fear, etched all over my face, and was waving me upwards with both hands and smiling in an encouraging manner.

With every fibre of my being, I was pulling on the swaying rope and willing my legs up, up, up. The race official grabbed my arm as I made the final last step up on to the solid rock top of the jebel. Instantly I fell to my knees. I could feel myself quivering with the fear, the effort – and the triumph. *I have just climbed an* actual *mountain.*

After a few breaths there on all fours, I allowed myself a smile of satisfaction and success. *I did it!*

People were passing me, patting me on the shoulder, saying words of encouragement.

That was the moment when I knew – I just knew – that I would finish the race. We still had three more stages to go, but as far as I was concerned, they were now conquered.

3

ROCKS, DUNES, HEAT

Marathon des Sables, 2013

'The person who comes last will get more glory!'

The long stage lived up to its name. Hours and hours of more of the same: rocks, dunes, heat.

Except this time we were making forward progress as best we could while the sun held the sky to ransom with a breathtaking sunset.

Fatigue was set deep in my bones. I could feel my blistered feet sticking to my filthy socks inside my trainers, damp with sweat. I trudged through grassy dunes, turning my head frequently to the right, observing as the sun sank lower and lower, throwing vibrant colours like flames simmering in the sky. The silky night encroached, dampening the dusky sunset colours down to intense dark blues, until finally it became deep black. Yet it was not dark. The moon, with a purity I had never seen before, shone bright, illuminating the landscape in a cool white glow.

How different the Sahara looked now.

In Camp the nights were dark and we huddled together in our tents, sharing stories of the day, joking, supporting and resting our weary bodies. Each evening we settled in for the night, hoping that our side of Camp faced the sun so that we could watch the spectacle of it setting.

There would be no sleep this evening, though. The long stage meant being in the Sahara at night, moving through it, and this was a totally different experience.

Without the familiarity of Camp around me, the Sahara became more vast, less hospitable, silent, isolating.

And yet, we were not alone, we runners; we had each other. A line of head torches stretched out in front of me, the small, slowly moving halos dotting the way through the dunes and stretching out for as far as I could see. There was no noise, just a profound silence all around us. The night seemed to lengthen and stretch out as the miles and my progress became slower.

It was difficult to know what the time was, as I had not worn a watch. I was running with my tent mate Pete, who was great company and had eyesight clearer than 20/20 vision. This came in quite useful when a dot on the horizon could be the first tent of a checkpoint, or just another rock. I would look with one eye closed, trying to focus with my one working contact lens; he would slightly narrow his eyes and then declare, 'Checkpoint.'

He was never wrong.

As we got closer to the stage finish line, we gathered a small group. There was no doubt in my mind that I wanted to do this stage in one go without sleep. This would mean a whole day off in Camp when I finally did wake up. But it was hard. The monotony of my food was taking its toll and despite my resolve to finish this stage as quickly as I could, my energy was very low. Coming into a checkpoint we met with one of the Hong Kong runners. His name was Jeff and he was extraordinarily tall.

We chatted as we trudged. He was a basketball player, and a hobby runner, so this race was his dream.

The three of us realised our strength lay in keeping together, pushing each other along in a group. My head torch was dimming, so I tilted my head downwards to capture whatever was just in front of my feet in the fading light. Kicking a small rock this many days in would be excruciating to my overtly sensitive and sore toes. We got into a rhythmic state of movement when all of a sudden I nearly fell over a leg.

I swivelled my head torch round and saw someone lying prone in the sand. 'You OK?'

'Urrrgh, leave me here. I don't care!'

'Come on, mate, get up.'

'No, it's fine.'

We all joined in the encouragement.

'You can do it!'

'Friend! Get up!'

'Hey, it's not too far now!'

'Last push. Get it done today, you can rest tomorrow!'

He lay there, looking up at the bright moonlit night. His head torch was blaring directly upwards into the night.

'The person who comes last will get more glory! I'll lie here, come last.'

He wasn't entirely wrong. Every day at the end of the stage, all of us would gather at the finish line at the cut-off time – and every day, making it just in time, one last weary runner made their wobbly way under the arch, closely followed by two camels and a convoy of race cars, lights blaring. Everyone cheered, clapping and whooping, giving them a hero's welcome, much more than the winner ever got with the whole field behind him still out on the race course. Here, everyone had made it to Camp, everyone could relate to the struggle, everyone was glad the person had made it safely in.

Behind them came the camels. The camels walked the whole distance, marking the back of the race along with their two camel handlers. This Camp camaraderie was very special, and each time watching the last person made me feel very emotional and happy to be there, starving, tired, caked in dirt – and part of something so unique.

'Come on! Get up!' I lightly kicked his leg with my foot.

With a grunt of resignation, he got up and joined us. Three became four.

48

His name was Krasse, he was Bulgarian, and he too was living his dream in this race.

••••

The darkness was pierced by a light on the horizon, blues and whites and a warm glow beyond. *Is this finally it?*

We had been moving for 16 hours. I did not want to believe that this could finally be the finish line for the long stage; the last hours had seemed never-ending, timeless, surreal.

'It *is* the finish! Let's run!'

Jeff was off, and he broke into a fast run, only to slow down after a minute because it was further away than it looked. We caught up and moved together towards the finish line, which slowly got bigger and bigger until, finally, we could see the words on the finish arch.

For the last few metres we broke into the fastest run we could muster, hand in hand, the four of us. Elated, we crossed the line together. We had started out as strangers from different parts of the planet, and yet here we were, all holding hands, hugging, smiling and sharing this unique moment as friends in the middle of the night in the middle of the Sahara Desert.

••••

I examined my feet. They were not as bad as some I had seen: a few minor blisters, some loose skin, redness. They ached like hell and were tender to touch. I used some iodine from a tent mate to try to clean them and propped them up as best I could, elevating them on my race bag, or even the tent poles for short periods of time. Most people's feet looked revolting. Some looked like they'd had a cheese grater taken to them and others like their toenails had been ripped clean out. I have a real aversion to grim feet and point-blank refused to go anywhere near the Doc Trotters tent. Stories of toenails being drilled into to relieve pressure and of deep infected wounds being cleaned out with stinging alcohol wipes made me feel a bit faint.

It was the fifth day and a lot of Camp had made it back in one stage. People were hobbling about, the Doc Trotters tent had a long queue, as did the communications tent, where a few basic computers had been set up so you could send an email. The atmosphere was light and optimistic. The dreaded long stage was done; we had broken the back of the race! Just the marathon stage to go to get our medal. Occasionally a ripple of applause would be heard and we knew that some more people had just crossed the finish line.

I tried to wash my clothes as best I could. Wearing my cut-off Tyvek suit, I cut a water bottle in half with my knife, and put some precious water in. I squashed in my socks, and refitted the top half of the bottle over, pushing to down so it overlapped the bottom half. I then shook it all hard as I could. The water immediately turned a dark cloudy brown. I held the bottle up and watched as the filthy water reabsorbed into the materials of the socks.

I squeezed it out and tried again with a bit more water, which seemed to clean a bit of the dirt off. I repeated this process with my top and hung it all up on the guy ropes by using my safety pins. I had to be careful with my water, tempting as it was to soak my clothes. The bottles are rationed for runners and if you want more, you will get a time penalty. You only get a couple of bottles at each checkpoint and more when you arrive back in Camp. It sounds quite terrifying, but the reality is there is enough to keep you hydrated, but not enough to wash your clothes in.

Life was incredibly simple here. Yes, I wanted to eat a 12-inch deep-pan pizza with a side of roast potatoes, and I could murder a pint of beer. I hadn't sat in a chair since I got here. (If you do not have a chair for a whole week you start to miss the simplicity of sitting in one, and wish you didn't have to sit all the way down on the floor.) Yet you made do with what you had – not a lot of things but an awful lot of new experiences.

Today was also the day I allowed myself one of my biggest rewards. Squirrelled away at the very bottom of my bag, in a tiny zipped compartment, was a note from Lily. I had held off reading it, using it as a little dangled carrot of encouragement to get me this far. Now I unzipped the compartment at the bottom of the bag, took it out of its small plastic ziplock bag, and unfolded it. She was a child and it was short, but I looked at her uneven child's handwriting with its simple message of love and encouragement, and smiled. This moment in my life could not have been further from Farnham, from my house, from my life as it was. I folded up the note and put it back in the little pocket to reread once I had my medal.

I was now down to the last few things to eat but despite a clawing hunger that had grown from my stomach and stretched itself right up to my chest, I could not face anything.

I had the option of a bag of seeds (very high calories, pack small, light, absolutely no fun to eat), a Camp muesli (*I'm never eating muesli again after this*) or a packet of Pop Tarts. The Pop Tarts had not been stress-tested for the rigours of the desert like the cheese and seeds; they had been a late entry to my desert food menu. They are not really good for you, have zero nutrients but are hugely calorific and don't weigh much. The silvery envelope containing them had held strong, but its contents had fared less well. Bashed and kicked around by being in the bottom of my rucksack for the week, the Pop Tarts had crumbled into pieces, and over the last few days remoulded themselves into a tight ball inside its container. Out of my three food options I went for the Pop Tart and tore open the silver packet.

The ball of crumbled sugary dough flew out and into the sand in front of my feet. I looked at it.

'That's a bit of bad luck,' my tent mate Glenn piped up.

I need the calories. I bent down and picked it up out of the sand. It was about the size of a golf ball and the sand had stuck all round, and though I was hungry to my core, it seemed repellent.

Dusting it off as best I could, I put it in my mouth and chewed gritty sand mixed with warm claggy dough. The occasional punch of oversweet sugar took the edge off. It was like eating the world's most miserable Ferrero Rocher.

••••

Though not at all nourished, I felt ready. Today was the last timed stage, the marathon stage. A full marathon, a further 26.2 miles, and at the end of this our medals.

Technically there would be one more stage tomorrow, but it would not be timed and it would be very short. Basically the last day would be us all walking out of a desert to a road to get on to a coach and back to the hotel; a place that, with all its soft furnishings and clean running water, still seemed like a distant dream.

Today was very much the last hurrah. Camp was in jovial and optimistic mood; we could all feel the temptingly close finish line. *Nearly there!*

There were babbles of conversations and laughter in the air; humorous insults and friendly goading between tents kept the mood sporting. Despite the gentle bragging, we all knew any one of us would be happy just to finish.

The time came and we made our way to the start line. People emerged from their tents – and how different we looked from that first day when we were all clean and mobile.

Now, what I saw was like some sort of zombie apocalypse. Many were limping. Everyone was filthy. We all had deeply ingrained dirt in our hair and in the creases of our skin, in the corners of our elbows, the folds of our fingers, our faces and necks. The grime had layered on. Once-clean clothes were now grey. Everyone had white tidemarks from sweat on their clothes, now hardened by the salt. Trainers taped together, beards grown, hair matted. I saw one guy with feet so swollen he had somehow obtained a pair of Crocs and was going to tackle the last stage in them. Already the sand was gathering through the holes and then sifting out again. I winced internally for him. However bad my feet were feeling now, they would not be as bad as his by the end of this stage. He had a long, painful day ahead.

'Is this thing getting further away or is it just me?'

Despite being in the same orientation every day, the start line seemed like a long way to go and that was before even beginning our race. My feet were stinging, I was painfully hungry and even now I'm not sure the condition of my hair will ever recover.

The now familiar sound of music blaring drew us in.

Patrick was standing on top of the Land Rover waving and dancing, like he had done every morning that week. He was beaming down at us like a proud father. He really cared how we all did and when he announced retirements – people who simply had not made it to today – he did get emotional. After announcing their numbers and names, we sang 'Happy Birthday' (again individually) to everyone who had a birthday that day (there were always at least two and some days there were more). Next, he gave us a speech.

Today, he said, was our day to enjoy, to take it all in – and he'd be seeing us next at the finish, where our medals awaited. The collective anticipation of the runners that had made it this far palpably went up a notch.

With one last blast of 'Highway to Hell' blaring from the speakers, we ran, jogged, walked and limped our way over the start line with considerably less panache and vigour than the first day, but with double the determination.

As we funnelled through the arch, the race helicopter swooped low overhead along the line of runners, which was already beginning to stretch out. We all cheered. And then, for one last time, into the dunes we went.

••••

Time takes on a strange quality in long races. It was hard to tell if I had been shuffling along for 20 minutes or an hour and a half. The landscape by now was familiar to me, but unlike before there were tiny signs of civilisation. Some telegraph poles on the horizon. A dirt road imprinted with tyre treads. Simple buildings dotted around, low-level and rudimentary, and most looking like they had been abandoned, but occasionally there was one with items visible – a bucket, some clothes, a curtain made from fabric in a glassless window.

I had been on the move for a couple of hours when I saw something on a sandy slope ahead. It was not a runner. Though I saw only its outline, I could tell it was moving differently.

Sometimes you think you can see things in the desert, but it is just the heat rising from the hot sand and distorting your vision. You can actually see the hot air; it shimmers and really does look like water. When I first saw this, I remembered old films from my childhood showing legionnaires seeing mirages and thinking they had found water in the hot, inhospitable desert.

What is that? Is it moving?

As I moved closer, the outline sharpened until it became clear. A boy on a bicycle, wearing a thick jumper.

A boy. On a bicycle. Wearing a jumper.

None of it made sense. Where on earth had he come from? I scanned around and could see no building at all in any direction. What use is a bike in the sand? Plus it was boiling hot. What could be worse to wear here than a woolly jumper?

As I approached, he held out his hand with a smile. I had nothing to give him, so apologised.

He smiled again and said, 'Allez! Allez!'

I carried on, and after a few seconds turned back to be sure I really had seen what I had seen. He was smiling and waving at the runners behind.

••••

I was weary, but there is something about knowing you are so close to the finish that helps you find the extra energy.

As I didn't own a sports watch, or think to buy a cheap one, it was difficult to gauge how much further there was to cover. I could sense I was near. *Surely.*

The race organisers have a tendency to do one of two things with the finish line: expose it so you can see it from miles away or hide the camp round a corner, just behind a jebel or sitting in a dip so you don't see it until it is very close. The first leaves you slogging through the desert looking at a finish that gets no closer. The second is equally painful; you spend so long hoping to see it, desperate to have eyes on it and wondering where it is, and when you do see it, you think it will still take time to reach.

I kept scanning and rescanning the horizon to get some idea of how much further I had to go. *Come on, where is it?*

Then suddenly, rising out of the heat haze in the far distance was the arch of the finish line. *I can see the finish! I am going to make it!* This sight had been such a huge goal of mine, my focus, my North Star, for the last several months, and now here it was, finally within sight.

We were strung out as runners, but a few of us whooped and pointed, and we all started running as fast as our legs could muster.

It was hard to tell but it looked about one kilometre away, so close! *The medal is so close!*

I had thought about this moment for so long before and during the race, what it would feel like to get there. In some more tired moments, the thought of reaching it had spurred me on and made me a little bit emotional, but now I was so nearly there and all I could think about was . . . *Just get it done. Then you won't have to get up and run again tomorrow. A shower! Some food!*

I suddenly became aware of a runner who seemed to be going in the wrong direction. We were all funnelling together on a narrow path that was a clear straight line in small sharp grey rocks all the way to the finish arch. Yet he was veering off to our left. I looked at him, noticing that he was leaning forward heavily and looking very unbalanced; he did not look right.

A momentary question about what to do flashed in my head. I looked at the finish and I looked at him. I started to run towards him. Two others did too.

He collapsed, straight on to the rocks.

The other two had got there quicker and he was unconscious.

Before I could do anything to help, someone released his distress flare.

It was huge and loud and shot up into the sky like a rocket, blazing a trail of light behind it.

It took me a second or two to register what was happening.

'Get help! Get help!!'

I started to run towards the finish line again. *JESUS CHRIST.*

As I was running as fast as my bleeding feet could take me, a staff car was driving towards him and passed by me.

'He fell! He's unconscious!' It was all I could say. The staff inside nodded acknowledgement at my words and then waved me towards the finish line.

It was about three hundred metres away and the arch was getting a tiny bit bigger with each few steps.

I kept thinking about the man who had fallen. He was so very close! Imagine being that close. Imagine a week of effort, then falling with the finish line in sight. I could hear the helicopter hovering behind in the near distance. I did not look back, and kept on looking and moving forward.

People lined the funnel, cheering, and the sun was beating down on to my arms, my legs. I felt nauseous and hungry in equal measure. This was it, the finish line! I saw Patrick clutching a medal in both hands, smiling. I returned the smile as I crossed the line and he placed a medal around my neck. I touched it with one hand and looked up to the sky.

I've done it. The Marathon des Sables. I've done it.

Rather than cry tears of happiness or feel extreme joy, I felt a mixture of relief and, more dominantly, a sense of knowing. Knowing that actually deep, deep down, I had always understood this moment would be mine. A tiny kernel of belief had been nurtured, trained and finally, after six long hard days, realised.

I was stronger than I had for so long allowed myself to believe. I had a strength and confidence that had been buried while I relied instead on alcohol and bluster.

A light had been shone to reveal an inner strength. Now I knew that the power and purpose of running would bring growth, more confidence and, definitely, more ultrarunning.

••••

I flew home from the Sahara a different person.

I got off the plane, got home and told my husband it was over.

My life was about to reboot. Things were changing. This was the new me – starting right now.

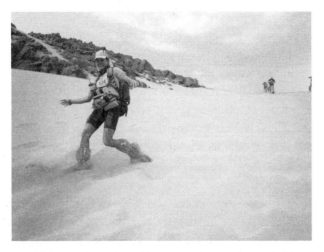

My first Marathon des Sables – there's no other race like it.

4

IT'S JUST ONE DAY IN YOUR LIFE

Thames Path 100, May 2014

'The sun is coming! You'll feel better when the sun comes up!'

The nerves are kicking in. One hundred miles. *ONE HUNDRED MILES?! Are you SURE?!* I take a very long blink and try to empty my mind of what is about to happen.

I am standing awkwardly on the periphery of a gaggle of people dressed in a variety of race vests, calf guards, running caps and jackets. A warm hum of anticipation and chatter ripples through the small crowd. There is not a single cloud in a blue sky and the sun is low and bright, its reflection glinting and sparkling off the River Thames.

We are in Richmond, on the outskirts of London, and this is where the Thames Path 100 is about to begin. One hundred miles along the path of the famous river, finishing in Oxford. If I make it, this will be the furthest I have run non-stop in one go.

It's probably too late to wonder if the previous three weeks have helped set me up for today or not.

Less than two weeks ago I ran the Boston Marathon and the week before that the London Marathon. While I took London relatively easily, Boston absolutely ruined my legs, because I gave it my all on the historic course. Now my post-Boston legs are the most sore my muscles have ever been after a race. I've not really done a lot in between, other than eating and trying not to think about running 100 miles.

I should probably eat something now, but cannot face the thought. Annoyingly, race day always seems to suppress my normally healthy appetite. When I should be eating a double breakfast, I can barely chew a bit of bagel.

Through the crowd there is a flash of bright orange. Then another! I recognise the exact hue of colour as this year's official Boston Marathon Finishers Jacket. My friends had turned up to see me off! Sophie Raworth, Ben Wickham and Jacquie Millett, a Wonder Woman of marathon running, have run here, all sporting the distinctive neon jacket, so I can see them from a mile off. We all ran Boston and friends like these are just the tonic in such moments, providing distraction and support in the last couple of minutes before the start.

We chat, a mix of soothing words from them as well as less soothing things like 'You are mad!' and 'One hundred miles is a very long way!

••••

It is a long way; so long that I could not actually look at the route. A few weeks earlier, I opened the race page on the website of the organisers, Centurion Running. The route flashed up on screen and was so big that it made Greater London look small. It wiggled its way across such a large proportion of England that I shut the image down immediately. *Sod that. That's ridiculous.*

I don't need to study it. I don't need to know what it looks like on a map.

It's 100 miles and my first attempt at the distance.

I never knew such events existed; that anyone would even contemplate covering such a distance on foot in one go. My first exposure to Centurion races came from my Marathon des Sables friend, Glenn. He was running one of the sister races, the South Downs 100 – as the title suggests, 100 miles along the somewhat hilly South Downs Way. Glenn is not the sort to tackle anything without gusto and he had started the race running along at a fair clip. It was his first centurion and in endurance events like this going out too hard means that things can unravel somewhat in the second half. I was to pace him from Mile 75; he turned up a little behind schedule, but looking very jolly. It became apparent very quickly, though, that he was in absolute bits. Because he sounded quite happy, I did not realise the extent of his pain. After about half a mile from our meeting point, he visibly winced stepping over a tree root, which stood about one inch proud off the ground. I realised that he was trying his very best to seem chirpy in front of me and that we were in for a very long night.

At one point the relentless hills of the South Downs became so much I fashioned him two walking sticks out of some tree branches to help him go both up and down the unforgiving hills. When we came into a checkpoint, there were several runners sitting in chairs, staring ahead. They looked hollow-eyed, hunched, broken. All of them said they would continue despite barely being able to walk easily. In that moment, slightly shocked to see what people willingly do to themselves, I vowed never to run 100 miles.

Crewing South Downs Way 100 was one of the longest nights of my life and included: yelling good morning to the sun in the dawn sky; coming up with the most insulting vulgar names imaginable for some sheep purely to keep our spirits up; and one absolute meltdown at Mile 92 when Glenn finally crumbled and actually said the words, 'I don't think I can do this.' To which I responded with my reserve tactic of losing my rag and telling him I had not spent the last night traipsing miles across the South Downs with his sorry arse only for him to give up 8 miles from the end.

'My car is at the finish line. I'm going there. You are coming with me, it's the least you could do after what we have just done.'

It worked: Glenn made it to the finish. After hours of listening to him muttering 'never again' over and over through the summer night, he called me up the next morning absolutely delighted, with virtually no recollection of the agonising miles shared and insisting I should run 100 miles myself.

Ultrarunners are both the best and the worst.

Seeing just how much pain everyone was in had put me right off. The thing about races, especially 100-mile races, is that you have to *want* to do them. After saying I never would, one day I woke up and out of nowhere decided that my time had arrived. That I wanted to find out what running 100 miles was like.

••••

So, there I was. Race Director James Elson had delivered a very sensible briefing, through which I paid minimal attention as I was still trying to empty my mind. I work best in a state of oblivion when it comes to ultrarunning. Some people like to pore over detail, routes, strategies. I choose to just tackle things as they face me: *it is what it is.* I had set myself the arbitrary time goal of completing the race in 24 hours – a time a fair amount of ultrarunners aim for – and firmly told myself, *it's just one day in your life.*

We were off!

The gaggle of runners started out. I waved goodbye to my friends. This race is as flat as 100-milers come in the UK and some front runners disappeared ahead quickly. I was going through a metal kissing gate when my watch beeped, alerting me to the fact I had run 1 mile.

Ninety-nine to go! said the voice in my head.

I shushed it quiet. *Empty thoughts, Susie, empty thoughts.*

Things ticked along without too much drama for the first 20 miles, and then, about 22 miles in, I suddenly became fixated with a minor niggle in my knee. It was all I could think about. *Why is it feeling like that now? It hurts! Is that a stabbing pain? I can't run 78 miles on this! Is it just going to get worse and worse? I'll never finish! What if I've broken it?!*

My thoughts started to spiral into mental hysteria.

The famous outline of Windsor Castle loomed ahead, poised above some trees at a curve of the river. This was around the marathon distance and I saw two more friends waiting for me.

One was the gloriously wonderful Rhalou, a carefree spirit and journalist, who held out a punnet of chips. The other was Simon Lamb, who I was also overjoyed to see, even though he didn't have any chips. A fan of ultrarunning, he was also my sports masseur and it was nothing short of a wonderful surprise to see both of them. I ate the chips while Simon pummelled my leg to work out any knots.

Rejoining the race after this little break my leg felt better and, fuelled by the chips, I felt better within myself. It is hard to tell if I was overthinking, or if Simon did indeed save my race: with so much time accompanied by just the thoughts inside your own head, you can make a drama out of virtually nothing. Either way, I felt improved.

The idyllic riverside town of Henley, famous for its rowing regatta, was just over halfway along the route. I had assumed I would reach this point in 10 to 11 hours and that I would generally be feeling OK, mentally and physically. Both assumptions turned out to be true and I was feeling quite buoyant coming into the checkpoint.

It was from here that I was allowed a pacer. This was something I was very much looking forward to – the distraction of someone to talk to and to help me pass the time. Hannah, my friend from a bootcamp class, was there, all grins and vim.

She chatted away to me while we made slow and steady progress. The Thames Path was still winding its way alongside the water, at times with buildings lining it. Grand homes with sprawling back gardens; tidy, well-kept hedges; and boathouses bigger than my own home. Other times it was open fields. The city of London had slowly thinned out, built-up urban areas giving way to the pretty towns in the home counties, in turn giving way to countryside. Trees hugged the trail, which was changing with the miles. At times it opened up, offering glimpses across open fields and train lines, only to narrow again so that all we could see were flashes of river through the trees framing either side of the trail.

The daylight slowly slipped away under the canopy, until we emerged after one enclosed section into the folds of the night. The darkness had a lulling effect on me. We were nearing the furthest distance I had ever run in one go: 100 km or 63 miles. The next big stop was Reading, which became a focus for me as an overwhelming sense of tiredness began to envelop me. Like a blanket popped on a cage to encourage a budgie to sleep, the darkness had a soporific effect. This was usually my bedtime, yet here I was plodding along a dark trail, deep into my first 100-mile race.

Hannah was doing her utmost to keep me with her by talking, asking me questions and chatting away.

My answers became more jumbled and shorter. My mind drifted off and away, craving sleep. Hunger pangs clawed at my stomach, yet there was nothing that seemed appealing to eat. My head sagged on my shoulders and my running feet turned into a shuffle, barely lifting off the ground. My eyelids drooped, narrowing in their fight against sleep. Sleep . . . sleep . . .

'WHOAH THERE!'

I could feel something grab at my arm. With a jolt I opened my eyes, trying to make sense out of the dark shapes ahead. They sharpened into familiar outlines of branches, tree trunks and a huge river about one foot away. I had fallen asleep running and nearly gone straight into the drink. Thank God Hannah was there – or who knows how that would have ended? It certainly woke me up.

We decided food was required and as we saw the lights of Reading bleeding into the night sky ahead a thought popped into my mind.

I had heard that the legendary ultrarunner Dean Karnazes once ordered a pizza during a long run. Could pizza be the answer here?

I have found generally in life that, no matter what the issue, pizza always helps.

It was worth a try. We called Domino's and placed an order. Then shuffled into the night, knowing that somewhere a pizza with anchovies (I was craving salt) was bubbling away in a pizza oven.

We came into a checkpoint – and there was the welcoming sight of Shaun holding a large Domino's box. He had collected it with his friend Carl and now he was to run with me for the rest of the night, all the way to the finish line. First, though, there were some minor complaints about having to sit in a car with a hot pizza and not being able to touch it.

I should explain that Shaun and I were in a relatively new relationship by this point, and I'd hesitated about asking him to crew me. I'd known Hannah for years, so her seeing me in my rawest form did not worry me too much, but a new boyfriend? That was slightly different. It would, I decided, be a good test of our relationship. Rather like the stress of a couple's first holiday, a first family Christmas, or being stuck in a traffic jam, exhausted and hungry – all distilled into a few hours.

Tempers can get sort of frayed out on the long run. Things can get most ungracious and unladylike too. It is what it is.

This was the time to be warts and all – and, frankly, I was utterly knackered and could not summon up any personality by this point. *He'll have to take me as I am, poor guy.*

I took two slices of pizza, rolled them up like a giant burrito and shoved them in my mouth. Pizza grease dripped down my chin.

'I think I need a piss,' I said through the chewing.

We waved goodbye to Hannah and Carl, and embarked on what would be, at that point, the longest and most testing night of my life – and quite possibly, despite 12 years in the army, Shaun's too.

The lights of Reading town centre woke me up a bit. Here, the Thames Path was no longer the soft mud of a trail but concrete, illuminated by halos of orange from street lamps. We ran alongside train tracks and through housing estates. It felt many times that we were off course and I repeatedly questioned if we were heading in the right direction, all sight of the river lost behind the suburbs. I jogged painfully past people who were heading home drunk and rowdy after a night at the clubs. There were a few boozy and jolly cheers. Running through Reading seemed never-ending.

If I was struggling as night drew in earlier, it was during the next section that the wheels totally fell off.

Mile 75 and onwards are a blur. Out of town, I was revisited by tiredness, this time more persistent, tougher to shake off. Stumbling around in the pitch-black for hours, field after field, gate after gate, was like being in some sort of infinite loop of mud and grass. Nothing seemed to change. With only the bob of my head torch casting a small circle of light ahead of me, I lost all sense of direction and all concept of time. My legs felt weak and unsteady underneath me as the same questions kept popping out of my mouth over and over. How far have we gone? Are we closer to the checkpoint? Do I need another wee?

'Seventy-eight miles.'

'A little bit, yes.'

'You just had one.'

Onwards we trudged. I was struggling to eat anything now and I had no energy left. Shaun was doing his best to get me to have something, yet the thought was nauseating. He was an absolute trooper: by this point I had fallen into a state of either stony silence or whimpering and whinging.

I was now overwhelmed; this is what ultrarunners call the death march. I was no longer able to run and it was all I could do to keep moving forwards. One foot in front of the other.

Onwards we went, my legs feeling like they were wading through treacle. *Why are these miles taking SO BLOODY LONG? When will we be OUT OF THESE HORRIBLE FIELDS?*

'Look!' Shaun pointed at where the orange blush of dawn was seeping into the night sky. 'The sun is coming! You'll feel better when the sun comes up!'

It had taken me an hour to cover just over 3 miles.

The daylight brought a renewed wakefulness. I managed to eat a bite of mooncake, a Chinese celebration cake that is small but absurdly rich in calories and sugar. I was feeling better, but my pace remained sluggish; I just could not get running again. It simply was not in me or my legs.

I went back to emptying my mind, closing in on the 91-mile mark, telling myself it was all about just staying upright and moving.

Shaun was having a conversation on the phone. I tried to tune out and just focus on making gradual progress, but then I heard something which made me fly into a rage.

'Yes, well, at this pace it will be about three to four hours . . . yes. Mile 91. See you at the finish!'

I'm sorry, WHAT? 'What did you just say?'

Shaun explained in his matter-of-fact way that he had been talking to my mother, who wanted to cheer me at the finish line, and that if we kept moving at this pace we would get to the end in three to four hours or so.

That was it.

The red mist descended.

'I am not doing this SHIT for another FOUR HOURS! ARE YOU JOKING?'

I could sense somewhere within me a door slam shut. Fortunately for me, that door was slamming shut on pain, not my resolve.

I started to run. No more death march for me; I simply could not stand this drawn-out agony any longer. The pain of my legs was eclipsed by the overwhelming desire for it all to be over – *and no way will that be before I got my hands on a One Hundred Mile Buckle.* I was utterly sick of the stupid Thames, its boring path and its relentless and ludicrous number of bloody gates. The Thames Path could get to fuck and I was going to finish this race as soon as possible.

Three miles after this running fury, I suddenly felt very wobbly indeed and nearly fainted. I ate another bite of mooncake, which enabled me to pick it up again. The miles passed quicker now and, invigorated by pure hatred for running . . . I ran.

I began to pass people; some gave me a wave or a shout-out as I passed, remarking on my pace. As I picked people off, this fuelled me further. I continued on my mission to get this over and done with.

I flew through the last checkpoint at Mile 95, refusing to stop. They clapped me as I went out; strangely the pace seemed more effortless now. The end was so, so close.

Twenty-four hours and fifty-eight minutes after I had started, there it was, the blue arch of the finish line looming ahead of me. I had done it! Punching the sky, I crossed the finish line, waving at my mother, who had just made it by minutes. Moments later, I fainted. Nibbles of mooncake and rage can take you only so far.

Shaun lifted my legs and I gently came round, feeling exhausted but jubilant. Unbelievably, the quickest miles across the whole 100 were the first three and the last three, set at a very similar pace.

••••

Carl, being the good egg he is, had come back to collect us. I was so tired I could barely speak and they practically carried me to the car.

I half-snoozed in the back seat.

'How was it?' I heard Carl ask.

'There was a whole bit in the middle where it was like getting your missus home from the pub drunk.'

At home they put me in the bathtub and switched on the shower. Still wearing all my race kit – race vest and number included – I let the water wash over me. I stank and so did everything I was wearing. The slice of pizza stuffed into my top pocket was absorbing water too.

Shaun came upstairs with a cup of sugary tea for me and to help me get undressed. He took in the scene of me broken and smelly, lying in a bathtub with a slice of Domino's in my clothing as the shower rained down – and smiled.

This is it, I decided. *He has done so much for me, and if he still fancies me after all this, he is definitely The One.*

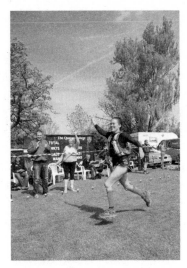

Twenty-four hours and 58 minutes later, here I am metres
away from the finish of my first 100-miler.

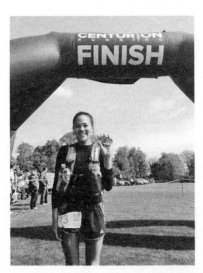

The relentlessness of the Thames Path was tough, but nothing would stop me
getting my hands on this One Hundred Mile Buckle.

5

EXPERIENCE WEIGHS NOTHING

Marathon des Sables, 2015

'The longer you are on your feet, the less time you have to rest. Things can start to spiral.'

It all seems familiar, yet different. What is it? As we travelled through South Morocco in the coach, I tried to put my finger on what exactly felt different and realised that instead of fear I felt nothing but excitement.

Two years later, I was back. A few things in the itinerary and Camp had been tweaked and improved, yet there was a familiarity about Camp. The two horseshoes of black tents; the rocks under the rug we slept on; the dry, dusty heat. Nothing was new or a surprise second time around, and I enjoyed being the one who had done it before.

I had returned for more with my boyfriend Shaun, selling it to him as 'one week's self-catering holiday somewhere hot, a bit of running!'

We signed up, and now, with somewhat less dedicated training and preparation, I was back in the Marathon des Sables Camp. I had run fewer miles this time around, but my approach was cleaner because the guesswork had been taken out. I had kept everything from the first time and now dug it all out, to be used again.

The event would be much the same as 2013, except this time I was equipped with something you cannot buy: experience. With several ultramarathons now under my belt and the knowledge of the landscape and mountains, and the fact that you cannot eat camping muesli with water every single day, I came into this one with a hearty dose of confidence – which weighs nothing.

Steve Dietrich greeted me like an old friend. He is the UK organiser of the race, fluent in French, and has worked on the Marathon since 2005. He has a handsome, kind face and a gentle, genial way about him, but he also exudes an air of wisdom and authority. In the years that he has been part of this event, he has seen it all. Seen the full range of desert ultrarunning – grim blisters popped on swollen feet, IVs applied to severely dehydrated runners – and listened to infinite frustrations and doubts, hugged those crying, talked countless people out of dropping out of the run. Every year he has returned to witness the determination, tenacity and, ultimately, victory of thousands of veterans of the race. For the UK runners, he's a safe pair of hands.

I have a lot of time for Steve and he has a lot of time for people. People gather around him pre-race, asking lots of nervous questions – about the race, the course, the logistics – question upon question. He listens patiently and takes his time with his answers, digesting what is being asked, giving it serious thought and responding honestly. When you are talking to him, he has a way of making you feel like you have his sole attention. He is a great race organiser and I have trusted Steve's judgement for so many more things in the years since.

For the race this time, I had some tips and tricks to help me. I had packed loads of food for Admin Day. My breakfast on the first morning was a vacuum-packed peanut butter and jam sandwich. I had varied my daily food, focusing on taste rather than a lighter weight. Rehydrated mashed potato was a game changer.

I had also been brutal with what I brought. Everything that went into my pack was heavily scrutinised. For every single item I had two questions.

'Is this absolutely essential?' If not, it did not come.

'Can it be lighter?' Consequently my pack this year was extremely light – 6.3 kg, just over the minimal kit requirement, and 3 kg lighter than my last effort at minimal packing in 2013. This would bring its own sacrifices, most of them to do with comfort – *but it's only a week*, I told myself.

••••

I felt very relaxed. Emily Foy, someone I had met on a tough race called Ring O' Fire in North Wales, was here too, as well as Paul, who was in my first race in 2013. A fantastic runner called Danny Kendal was also in my tent. He was an elite runner, and I thought I had done well with my pack weight. Sitting next to him in camp on Admin Day brought a whole new level to cutting weight, though. I watched as he produced a pair of scissors and trimmed the labels off his clothes, and cut away extra pockets and unused bits of straps on his bag. We had to carry €200 with us, and he had one €100 note and five €20 notes, and was now looking for someone to swap the €20s for two €50s or a simple €100 instead. The only thing he had not scrimped on was food.

'Got to keep eating,' he told me with a sage nod.

I had no specific plans for this race, although I did feel like my fitness was pretty good. I had a simple goal: to walk less than I did a few years ago. The course is different every year, so going for a faster time is not a realistic target.

This year marked the race's 30th anniversary and we were told to be in for a surprise on the long stage. I do not like surprises and when we discovered that the long stage would be one of the longest in the history of the race at a juicy 57 miles, ripples of uneasy anticipation worked their way around Camp. I pulled out the roadbook and consulted the cartoon map, turned the page to the long stage section and saw that there was a huge stint of sand dunes in the last third. *At least we'll be getting our money's worth.*

By now, though, I had found peace in the fact that there are some things you can control and others you can't. The prospect of the long stage did not bother me too much. I was going to focus on trying to eat better, move slightly faster, and not forget to take my salt tablets.

I could not possibly have predicted how the race would unfold.

••••

On Day 1, Shaun and I set off with the aim of keeping together for the race. He is a strong runner, stronger than me, but we decided that was the plan and off we set, adopting a steady pace while people around us raced off ahead. It was his first time at the event and despite his experience as a soldier in hot desert environments, surviving all sorts of troubling events in very basic living conditions, he was about to discover that running through the Sahara self-sufficiently is a very different experience.

Day 1 was as expected, little bits of everything; all our tent mates came home in one piece and we shared our stories from the day. We were relaxing into the race.

I was happy and energised, and ready to take on my race nemesis on Day 2: Jebel El Otfal. The mountain.

The day started like any other. The skies were calm, clear and blue, and there was not much wind to pick up the sand and swirl it in the air. Knowing how the mountain had frozen me in fear last time, I went into the day in the same way that I deal with a lot of things that make me uncomfortable: by clearing my mind and simply doing my best not to think about it until it's happening.

The sun rose higher in the sky and the temperature rose too. Degree by degree, it crept up. Our sweat was evaporating on our foreheads before it had time to trickle down our faces. Today we were taking on the shorter course (18 miles) and had already covered a high rocky peak when Shaun became quiet. We went through a checkpoint, greeted by Doc Trotters, our name tags pulled out on their retractable elastic bands and stamped to show we had passed through. We were reminded to take our salts.

Shaun stopped and wandered in a different direction to the course, looking for shade by one of the Land Rovers that make up the checkpoint.

'You OK?'

'Bit hot.'

We had trained in a heat chamber for this race, every couple of days going into the small room in Kingston University to run or cycle at a temperature of 38°C. We had come as prepared as possible for this heat. The checkpoint sat a couple of kilometres away from the huge mountain ahead of us, ominously filling the view. Between the row of Land Rovers making up the checkpoint and the mountain was the long, cracked hard ground of a salt flat.

After a short break at the checkpoint, we pressed on. There was no breeze at all as we moved across the salt flat. Shaun started to slow, but I was keen to get up and over the mountain with minimal fuss, not wanting to dwell on the climb, and completing it as quickly as possible. We came out of the salt flat and, after posing for a photo, arms spread wide and smiling to the camera, things unravelled. Shaun started to feel unsteady. There were no further checkpoints ahead, just the finish line on the other side of the huge mountain. The memory of the poor chap who had wobbled until he fell flat on his face, knocking himself out, flashed into my head.

This was the most technically difficult part of the entire course, between us and the finish line, and Shaun was looking very peaky indeed. Any trepidation I had about the approaching mountain was now buried under the more pressing difficulty of getting up and over in the heat of the day.

The next hour passed with a lot of encouragement from me, a lot of holding on to rocks, a lot of moments where Shaun looked like he might puke, and a lot of silent grit on his part. All of the mental preparation I had made to help me over this moment – knowing that though I had conquered it before I would still probably be frightened – fell to the wayside as we made it up and over the thing patiently and methodically as a team. Progress was slow and once we crested the top the sun was at its highest, blazing down. There was no shade anywhere.

Slowly we picked our way downwards until finally we made it back to the welcome shade of Camp.

Tent mates Gordon and Rob tried to encourage Shaun to visit the medical tent, to no avail. He was determined to tough it out.

By Day 3, Shaun and I had decided not to run together, because he said he needed to take it easy.

The whole tent watched as he drank some water and then immediately threw it up on his own feet. Still he refused to go to the doctor, worried that he would be pulled from the race.

Unsure of what to do for the best, we finally decided that there were enough people out on the course to turn to if things went south for him, and there would be no point both of us walking.

Off I went, tagging on along with Emily, who is a far stronger runner than myself. We ran solidly that day; I felt strong and well within my comfort zone. The sand dunes did not feel so big or the climbs so gnarly, and the heat was more bearable. By the time we crossed the line, I had leapt up the leader board with Emily. That was a turn-up for the books and I was buzzing! The great feeling did not last, though, because when Shaun arrived back at Camp he looked very pale.

He was feeling worse than the day before and still vomiting. Recovery is difficult in this race; you have only what you have carried with you. The longer you are on your feet, the less time you have to rest. Things can spiral.

••••

Day 4 was the dreaded long day and it was indeed long, really long. We made our way to the start and I watched as Shaun walked to the line. There was a resigned air about him, something not unfamiliar to me – that sense of dread you have knowing things are about to start hurting, knowing that you will keep going as long as there is a possibility of finishing. It's a mixture of wanting to keep face, of pride, of fearing failure, of wanting to make the finish line – a lot of different emotions. I felt for him, but he's an adult and he had made his choice to continue.

We said our goodbyes and once again Emily let me tag along with her. We set off at a steady pace. Today, when the course was so very long, our goal was to keep running for all the runnable bits – the flats, the downhills and shallow dunes. The only place we would not try to run would be up a large dune or up a mountain. How long could this last for me? Emily is a superb runner, she could take this in her stride, but I was not so good on elevation. My plan was to try to cling on for as long as possible.

As we kept going, I worried about Shaun: every time there was a tough section and some high dunes, and when the sun rose high into the middle of the sky, I thought about him. The sun was unforgiving, shining down on every nook of the desert, heating up everything it touched. There was simply no shade, just fiery heat.

I was also worried because today had the dreaded ascent of the Jebel El Otfal again – two ascents in one race. This time we would be climbing up it in reverse, which meant a gradual slow climb up and over giant rocks, which are hot to touch and overbearing.

Emily and I slogged it out; keeping momentum was difficult because there was no obvious path. In parts, you have to find your way through, choosing the best way to navigate around large rocks, sometimes climbing, sometimes squeezing around, sometimes watching those in front of you, noting their choices and how well they manage.

As we made progress upwards, I started to feel anxious about the top of the mountain and what was waiting over the other side. We both knew what we were about to encounter there: the highest point in the race, the part that needed ropes to climb, the very point where a slight glance had triggered my vertigo and paralysed me with fear only a couple of years before. We would be running directly down the opposite way I had climbed up before. Once we had reached the summit, there was simply no way to avoid looking directly at it.

'We are just going to not think and run.' Emily's voice was soft, but there was also a finality to it. I internalised a growing panic.

The huge rocks made way for the last bit of the climb. As we neared the pinnacle, the mountainside was littered with small, sharp rocks. A helicopter whirled and buzzed overhead. I could not yet see over the top to the view and the drop had not yet revealed itself. My steps naturally slowed in anticipation and dread.

'Come on! Let's keep going!'

Oh god. I deliberately looked down at my feet rather than up to see what lay ahead. I was a half-step behind Emily. 'Emily, I'm not sure . . .'

Before I could finish my sentence, she grabbed hold of my hand and pulled me over the crest of the mountain.

Gravity had a hold of me. The shock of what was happening blended in with the simple reaction of just trying not to fall. My legs kicking out in front of me, feet sinking into the sand, one after the other in quick succession over and over and over. Instinctively I threw my arms up to help balance, eyes wide, scanning where my feet were landing, quickly sidestepping hidden jagged rocks. I held my breath and tried to stay upright.

Emily was in front, arms out steady and open as she ran down this enormous mountain dune. She looked effortless, controlled. 'WHOOOAAA!'

About halfway down, the gradient slightly reduced. I felt a bit more in control of my descent and, with a rush of adrenaline, I realised that perhaps this was not terrifying and that perhaps, just perhaps, this was a moment of a lifetime, one to be savoured.

'WHOOOAAA, WE ARE DOING IT!' I yelled back.

With my arms still flailing around, and still trying not to let gravity win, still avoiding pointy rocks, I felt a huge rush, like stepping off a rollercoaster or a huge, happy shock.

The gradient softened further as the mountain eased into the desert ground, still downhill but runnable. Now feeling more in command of my legs, I ran hard to catch Emily: elated, exhilarated, excited.

'Controlled falling,' Emily called it. We continued, still running. The sun started to sink lower, the temperature began to cool and evening set in. Onwards we ran, in step, making progress through the miles. The elite runners passed us as dusk fell. We cheered Danny Kendall, who was having a great race.

We passed through a large checkpoint. Usually on a long stage some runners choose to sleep overnight and extra tents are set up for this purpose. The race organisers had decided, though, that this would be a little different to other years. There was all manner of temptations to keep us entertained, celebrating this special 30th edition of the race.

There was a tiny cup of mint tea for all runners. A sweet refreshing drink that meant a welcome few calories for us. Only one each, though; they were strict! An array of deckchairs was dotted around, all facing a glorious view. More inexplicably, a small jazz band was playing. Light trumpets and the rat-tat-tatting of a brush drumstick filled the dimming night sky. Patrick had hired an actual jazz band to come out to the middle of the southern Sahara and entertain us. Party lights were dotted around. It was surreal – and wonderful. And intended to be a reward for getting this far, but it was more like torture having to pretend we did not actually want to sit in a deckchair, listening to music, drinking sugary mint tea. We did not stop and pressed onwards.

More running. My legs were feeling very weary and within myself I was feeling very tired. I had not eaten a meal all day and it was becoming difficult to concentrate on anything. A deep shadowy night fell, swallowing all the light. We started to fall into step with a third female.

Initially we skirted around each other, leapfrogging each other politely, respectfully giving each other space, while knowing we were in the same race. After an hour or so like this she called out to us: 'Hey! I'm Holly!'

'Hey! How you doing?'

So two became three. There is strength in numbers in these tough sections. We all fell into step, running, running, running. I couldn't believe I was still running.

My head torch was weakening and I became mesmerised by the dimming circle of light bobbing around ahead of my feet. Occasionally I looked up and realised that I had dropped back. Then I had to work so very hard, putting effort into each step to stay with Emily and Holly. In a mix of dim night and foggy head torch, I was struggling to tell if I was running uphill or downhill or flat.

Finally, we came in to the last checkpoint. Now there were just 6 more miles to go to the finish line. We had completed 51 miles. Holly reached into a side pocket of her rucksack and pulled out a small bag, and within it were three Peanut M&M's.

'One each,' she said.

This gesture was so generous. This should have been her treat for herself, and she had perhaps saved them for this long stage. After the usual Britishness – *we couldn't possibly, no, no, you have them* – Holly insisted. Emily and I took a single M&M each. 'They melt, but stay solid under the sugar shell,' she told us.

As it dissolved in my mouth, it tasted like a dream – a sugary, sweet, nutty dream.

Fuelled by the sweets and the power of each other's company, we charged home in the longest stage ever. We crossed the line hand in hand, so the race organisers gave us all joint 10th place.

I was so tired, so spent, and I could not believe that I had run as hard as that for that long in that environment. I thanked them over and over. If not for them, I would have started to walk a long time ago and would still be out there. Running with stronger people, positive people like Emily and Holly, had shown me that I was capable of more than I thought, that I was stronger, faster and more determined. Once again, the Sahara Desert had taught me a lesson.

••••

Waiting for Shaun was painful. The sun had risen and people were coming back all night and all morning. Camp babbled with quietly content people, happy to have got the long stage done. Dusty and weary, people just kept on coming over the finish line, some limping, some jubilant, and none of them Shaun.

I waited and waited, out in the sun by the finish until someone from the race told me to get in the shade.

'It's not good for you to be out in this sun all day.'

I went and sat under the shade of a giant inflatable teapot by the finish line. Like the jazz checkpoint from the previous night, this was another slightly surreal element. The race was sponsored by a tea company that year, and a giant teapot came with the Camp. Moving round with us, it was huge and you could see it from miles away, popping up at the start and finish line. Now I leaned on it, on the shady side, keeping my eyes on the horizon.

Midday came and went.

We were now within a couple of hours of the cut-off.

Sir Ranulph Fiennes crossed the line. The legendary explorer was 74 years old and had developed the dreaded ultrarunners lean as he walked, curved over to one side. He was slow but continued with a tenacity and resolve that you would expect from someone who has survived expeditions in some of the most arduous climates.

Still no sign of Shaun. Most people were back. Stragglers were few and far between.

With every single person that appeared through the heat haze, I sat up and stared hard at the form, trying to find familiarity in the walk, the shape of the body or the colour of the clothes.

I asked people as they had crossed the line if they had seen him.

One person had. 'He's out there. He doesn't look great, but he is still moving.'

Another hour passed.

Another figure appeared on the horizon. I squinted, trying to take in the colour of the hat. *Is it yellow? Shaun has a yellow hat on. Is it him? Is that yellow?*

As the figure moved slowly but steadfastly towards the finish line, *it is him! It is!* I ran out of the shade of the teapot towards him.

He was not one to make a big fuss, but when he got back to our tent, tentmate Rob sacrificed valuable calories and gave him one of his recovery shakes. It helped.

Then Shaun slept. When he woke, he talked lightly of trudging painfully for miles, of trying to stay focused, of passing out in the dunes, of someone trying to set off his distress signal. He had been toughing it out for hours and hours and hours.

'You don't have to do this, you know.'

'I know. I have my reasons.'

We were having completely different races. He was really happy to hear that I had done well and the whole tent was relieved there was only one stage left.

••••

The elite field were announced that evening. People came round to the tent and called out a number. The elites leave an hour after all the main runners, when the day is slightly hotter. The organisers hold back the faster runners so that they do not blitz through the course more quickly than checkpoints can be set up. Someone popped their head in our tent.

'Danny Kendall? You are in the elite field, start at 10 a.m.'

This was expected – he had been running with the front runners each day – and we all clapped.

'Susie Chan? You are in the elite field. Start at 10 a.m.'

Say what?!

Emily and I went over to the noticeboard, scanning the list of finish times. Emily was well in time with a strong first two days, but I had just made the elite cut. One hundred people would leave after the main field of over 1300 runners and I was among them. I was both thrilled and nauseated. I had only just made it, coming in at 98th.

I did not want to be last out of the elites.

I stood on the start line of the marathon stage with a renewed focus, a refreshed perspective and all of my determination funnelled into this last day. This week could not have been further from the week I had anticipated in my head. Shaun, a much stronger runner than me, had been through the wringer and was now clinging on to the race by the skin of his teeth. That morning, rested and managing to keep some food down, he reassured me that if he could get through the long stage, he could get through today. Everyone had the same feeling: just one more day. It had been the longest race in the history of the Marathon des Sables and we were not going to let one final, pesky marathon get in the way of what we had worked so hard for. Everyone was going to finish.

To the familiar sound of AC/DC blaring out, we watched as the main field set off. I found myself remembering what it had felt like for me a couple of years before: all the emotions of relief on that last day, the hunger, the joy, the pain, and ultimately embracing what was about to happen and knowing that I was so close to the finish.

Those were feelings familiar to all of us and, whether shuffling or running, everyone on the final day is desert-filthy and determined. The medal awaits.

We waved and cheered off the main start, then for an hour we had nothing to do but wait and watch as Camp was taken down and taken away on one truck after the other, driven onwards to be rebuilt at the finish line.

This was a flat stage, so I was going to run with every fibre of my being to that finish line. Somehow, I had made it into the elite start line and I wanted to do it justice. This had to be my best effort.

Once again running next to Emily, we charged off out from under the white arch and straight over the small dunes, directly into a sandy headwind.

All I could think about was running no matter what. *I did it before, I can do it again.* Through checkpoints with minimal fuss, we kept going, kept running. As we made it through the miles, we passed people who had left before us, and it was not too long before I saw the familiar yellow hat of Shaun. He looked considerably better than the previous day and was advancing steadily with a small group of people, ahead of the last-place camels. Buoyed by seeing him, I kept on the charge.

There was something fabulous about passing people who clapped and cheered us. I had never been in this position and lapped it up gleefully, each bit of encouragement feeding me and making me feel a tiny bit stronger. The miles seemed to pass more effortlessly than on previous days; the course threw a few dunes at us, but it was generally flatter and seeing people the entire way certainly helped. This felt much more like a race – and so we raced.

When we saw the finish line of the Marathon des Sables ahead, we picked it up even more. A French man was suddenly running next to Emily and me, grinning from ear to ear: 'Allez! Allez!'

How different it was this time. No dramas, just delight. I was full of energy. Emily ran faster, I ran faster.

'Allez, allez, allez!' we all chorused together, racing towards the finish.

I felt light on my feet, fast, like I was flying.

••••

With my medal around my neck, I felt my race was not over. I dumped my pack back in the tent and returned to the finish line to wait. It is a joyous place to be. Emotions run high as you see people realise their running dream by finishing the race. Tears, hugs, exhaustion, cheers, medals – what running is all about.

I clapped, watched and waited, chatted, watched and waited, wondered where he was.

Steve came up to me to congratulate me on my race, all kind eyes and warm smiles. 'Steve, do you know where Shaun is?'

Steve came back to me. 'Word on the course is he is on for a negative split!' he joked. Another warm smile. [If you're wondering, a negative split is the strategy of running the second half of a race faster than the first.]

I started to walk back out down the course.

After about a kilometre, I found a rock to sit on.

The yellow hat appeared on the horizon, his familiar form.

I ran to greet him, arms aloft waving in happiness! *We're going to do it — both of us finish the race!* Hand in hand we headed to the finish, breaking into a run in the last 100 metres.

Emily and our tent mates were cheering, friends were watching at home via the webcam, and we finally did what we had planned: we crossed the finish line together.

After a huge hug Shaun put his hands on his legs and started to get on his knees.

Oh Jesus, don't puke up here.

And then, on one knee, he produced a ring.

'It's what kept me going,' he said.

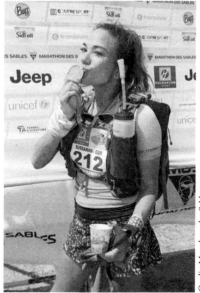

My second Marathon des Sables. I sold this to Shaun as a self-catering holiday somewhere hot, with a bit of running...

6

SNAKES AND LADDERS

Jungle Ultra, Peru, 2016

*'I cried at the start line. I cried with a mixture of
exhaustion and fear.'*

I am falling. This one is a big one: sliding downhill with my
arms flailing, trying to find anything to grab to stop the slide.
I get hold of a plant, which immediately crumbles in my
grasp. I try another branch, which stabs me in the palms with
thorns. I continue to slide.

What if I never stop sliding and am lost forever?

A third attempt on a small stump gives me enough to halt my
undignified slide. Lying here winded and caked in mud, I am
sweating profusely in the humidity. I am bleeding from scratches,
and within seconds I can also feel an army of ants crawling,
biting and sticking to my clammy skin. Under my clothes, they
itch and nip.

I hate it here. A tiny part of me wants, out of sheer tiredness,
just to keep on sliding. I simply don't care anymore. *Running is
stupid. This is it,* my inner voice says. *This is what it finally feels like
to reach your limit. You're done.*

This is new. In the past I have experienced everything
during races, from fury to exhaustion to questioning my life
choices, but I have never felt like this. This is despair. Utter
despair. I have nothing left, no desire to continue, to run, or
even to stand up.

I have spent the best part of an hour trying to work my way upwards through the thick vegetation. At what point does a bush become a tree? I have never seen plants so big, or leaves that are metres wide and tall. There is growth everywhere I look – all around me, covering the floor of the jungle, as far up as the eye can see, blocking out a lot of the light. Plants are wrapped around other plants. And everywhere is alive. The prospect of giant spiders appearing terrifies me.

In the jungle you get the distinct impression that a thousand bug eyes are on you at any given moment. Looking out from under logs or from a great height. The ones that want to bite you are terrifying to an arachnophobe like myself. I try not to think about the biting spiders.

In the slippery mud, I can get virtually no purchase underfoot. I am climbing, climbing, and climbing up what feels like the sheer savage face of the rainforest. This is more of a fight with nature than running. This is vegetation with meat on its bones.

Physically I am shattered; this is beyond tedious and just staying focused on moving forward is itself a mental battle. I am making painfully slow progress and now, finally, with the top in sight, I lose my footing.

I am back where I started, having fallen all the way back down. Weighed down by my bulky rucksack, I lie there like an upturned beetle contemplating how on earth I, a normal person, have ended up here. It was not that long ago I was sitting at a desk making a mental note to buy a tin of Whiskas for Sinbad, my cat, on the way home. I am now thousands of miles from civilisation, from my small but cosy house in Surrey.

I look up into the canopy of trees above me. I can just make out small patches of sky through the dark green ceiling, layer upon layer of branches and foliage. Everything is damp – my clothes, the air, my spirits. Every breath of air smells like earthy mud and wet leaves. I can taste salt in my mouth and feel my skin itching from hundreds of tiny painful cuts. Somewhere deep in the Amazon rainforest, many miles south of Lima, Peru,

I wail: *Ahhhhhhhhhhhhhhhhhhhh!* A proper self-pitying wail from the bottom of my stomach. No one hears.

And this is the fourth day – the fourth day of this utter, total bullshit.

I am about to be taught a valuable and extremely painful lesson. A lesson so severe I will emerge vowing to never, ever, ever set foot back in a jungle.

••••

Wind back several months, and my partner Shaun and I were channel-hopping when we stumbled across a documentary. Suddenly on the screen was someone running in the jungle, wearing a race bib. A chap called Richard Parks, taking part in a race called Jungle Ultra. It didn't look too bad. Sure, the terrain looked muddy in parts, and there were river crossings, but the whole episode reeked of adventure.

At this point, I should admit that I'm terribly impressionable. TV adverts work brilliantly on my simple mind: all I need to see is a pizza box and I want pizza. Such impressionability has been a bit of a hindrance overall, to be honest.

Right then, on TV, the race looked relatively manageable. Only in hindsight did I conclude that the camera crews could not possibly have accessed huge parts of the course, or seen the misery – as well as the true wonder – that the jungle has to offer.

The format for this race is similar to the Marathon des Sables: multistage racing. Five days of running with a finish line edging closer to the Amazon Basin and the relative comfort of a small town, Pilcopata. It takes place in June, neither the wettest nor the hottest time of year for a jungle. In between the starting point and the end is 250 kilometres (155 miles) of the odd dirt road, endless foliage, streams and rivers, and a lot of elevation. We would start off around 14,000 feet up – the typical height for jumping from a plane to skydive is 10,000 feet. Starting at altitude is unusual, meaning that the race is a net downhill run!

The problem with looking at race statistics as a guide to the race, though, is the element which you cannot define with numbers – and that is the terrain. I was to discover that running just one mile can be very different in a jungle.

Another unusual feature of this race is the different daily mileages. Not only do the days get longer as the week progresses, they get more difficult. You start at high altitude, in summer, where it is warm. The weather is calm, but as you move lower and through the course, conditions get hotter and more humid, more 'jungly'. This coupled with fatigue and hunger, which both increase day upon day.

The last day is the longest stage. Even at the time I recognised this was not ideal, but as with most races you can only go on the facts presented to you – and on paper it seemed manageable. The format was familiar, though it was somewhere new, a new environment to run in. And it looked great in the pictures!

There was also a new race director, the enterprising Kris King. We chatted before the race and he made it sound more like an expedition, like nothing I had ever experienced.

To be frank, the prospect of giant spiders was seriously putting me off. I generally swerve sheds, outbuildings, sitting on logs in the woods and the like – any situation, in fact, which could increase the chances of me meeting a spider. I hate them. Being from the home counties in the UK, I didn't really have too much concept of jungle animals, either. But this was the jungle, the real deal, full of predators and poisonous things.

However, Shaun was very keen I did not dwell on the risks or any worst-case scenarios. And it's true I'm of the mind that such thinking is not really very helpful in the world of ultrarunning anyway. So, feeling a little bit responsible for putting him through the Marathon des Sables, I agreed. *It's only running, right?*

••••

Like the Marathon des Sables, the Jungle Ultra is self-sufficient. Runners carry all the things needed to survive the rigours of a week in the jungle.

This includes all food, which makes up most of the weight; a basic first aid kit, just enough for the most rudimentary care; a sleeping bag; and, if there is space left, any luxuries you might want. Luxuries are anything in addition to the mandatory kit list and something you consider worth lugging around as extra weight for the week. The definition of luxury in this scenario is broad. Something as simple as a clean change of socks, an inflatable pillow or a note from a loved one can change your day. Again like the Marathon des Sables, all these things are packed in a rucksack to be carried with you every step of the way, so it is crucial to keep weight to a minimum.

The only difference between the Marathon des Sables and the Jungle Ultra is that all the things in your rucksack need to be thoroughly waterproofed. A simple step – and one I neglected out of ignorance, from the start. It was the root of nearly all my misery during the week. The jungle is hot, but unlike the desert this is not dry heat. When everything is wet through, it stays wet – and weighs so much more.

I did get some things right. Experience has taught me not to take a single thing that is not necessary. Apart from cheese. Nothing like a nibble of Parmesan to cheer you up after a long day's running. That and some packets of Chewits Xtreme were my only luxuries. Tasty food is vital in these races.

Aside from food, the biggest and heaviest bit of kit we also had to carry became my comfort and nemesis in equal measures: a hammock. Each night when we had completed that stage of running, we simply pitched our hammocks and went into recovery mode: rehydrated whatever dehydrated race fodder we had bought, ate some food and replenished some of the calories burned that day – and then slept.

Hot and cold clean water was provided by the race organisers. The simple life.

••••

I was looking forward to going to an entirely new continent and an entirely new environment. Shaun and I flew into Cusco, a vibrant historic city where the friendly locals dress in brightly coloured fabrics and the alpacas wear tassels. The city is a dreamy blend of history and culture old and new, surrounded by mountains. It's photogenic in every direction. They know how to throw a street party and the whole city has a happy buzz. It's a fantastic place, welcoming and warm in both senses of the word. Modern fine dining cuisine next to the local delicacy, guinea pigs. You feel safe meandering the narrow streets. No wonder it's popular. It's one of the hubs that people visit on their way to Machu Picchu. The whole city is a celebrated UNESCO World Heritage Site.

The bars, hotels and restaurants were superb. We found a pizza restaurant on our first day there. The pizza was cheap, fresh and delicious. We sat on a balcony overlooking the Main Square and took in the city beneath us. There was a succession of bands; there was always some sort of music coming from somewhere. The city was so vividly culturally rich and new to me that I could have stayed there for weeks and not got bored. Unfortunately, we were there for only a couple of nights, in order to acclimatise to the altitude.

Cusco stands at an altitude of 10,990 feet and is within the range considered 'moderate danger' for altitude sickness. I had never been this high up before and felt like I was breathing through a straw. Just walking up one flight of stairs on the day we arrived had been a little bit chewy. There are bowls of coca leaves around the hotels and immediately upon arrival we were offered coca tea. This apparently helps mitigate the tight-chest feeling created by the thin air. All things considered it wasn't too bad and with the overall descent of the race from the get-go, I did not let this detail bother me.

After two nights in Cusco, we all piled into minibuses and travelled north-east for around six hours, rattling around the tinny vehicles as tarmac roads quickly turned into potholed dirt tracks. This was the first time meeting our fellow runners. Most of us came from the UK and we were in high spirits. If there were any nerves in the group, they were undetectable. There was a lot of chatter about race kit, our time in Cusco and past races, which eventually made way for quiet curiosity as we watched the landscape turn from city to rural to wilderness.

We finally reached our destination, a few thousand feet further up than Cusco: the Manú National Park. This is cloud forest, so named because the jungle sits at high altitude with persistent cloud cover. The whole national park is a huge conservation area, richly biodiverse. Nearly the same size as Portugal, it is thousands of square miles and like Cusco it is protected by UNESCO. Large areas are restricted, home to indigenous tribes. Access to these regions is allowed only for research. In areas that are non-restricted, sustainable tourism is allowed, including this race.

It was an extraordinary place to be and here, for the first time, we camped out. This was the day before the start and Kris, the race director, delivered a full and edifying race briefing. He told us to try not to get bitten by snakes, not to cross the path of the main jungle predator (the jaguar) and not to touch certain plants (details I instantly forgot because they all look rather similar in a jungle). He also advised us to tie down our rucksacks or even to sleep with them inside our hammocks to stop snakes getting inside and monkeys stealing them. He paid particular attention to safety in water, given that there were numerous rivers to pass through, and suggested this would probably be our greatest risk. Some of the rivers could be fast-flowing and he told us what to do if we thought we might be drowning. We all had trackers with a distress button and were advised to do our best to get to the side of the river and, if needed, sound the alarm. Ideally, we should try to stay with others for river crossings for safety. This was a far cry from pedestrian race briefings of the past about road safety and course cutting. A slide presentation included the route of wiggly lines through a rainforest with no notable landmarks at all, how to operate your tracker in an emergency, the physical signs to be aware of for heat stroke. He ended the whole thing on a picture of a butterfly to 'make you all feel nice.'

Unbeknown to us, weeks and weeks of work had gone into getting this race ready for its start line. The small race team are very ecologically conscious and this event is the biggest in this remote corner of the globe. The team relies heavily on local people to help set everything up and a fair amount of the race entry goes back into these small communities. The route itself is never exactly the same year on year, as it is cut fresh into the jungle. It takes eight locals eight weeks to do this; they set up camps as they go and work their way through the entire route, hacking away with machetes. Six months after the race is over, there is no trace of the route; the jungle quickly reclaims these temporary trails as its own.

The route is not exclusively fresh jungle trails, though. Mercifully, there are some stretches through farmland and, now and again, you take in dirt roads. Somewhat less mercifully, there are 70 river crossings, which are accomplished in a variety of ways: mainly on foot where vaguely passable, but if the river is too high or turbulent, dinghies and zip wires are manned by the locals to assist runners across.

••••

Day 1. In clean race kit, looking fresh and smelling vaguely presentable, we assembled at the start line. A small but keen group of like-minded individuals, all shiny and spirited at the prospect of a five-day adventure. I recognised a couple of the group from the small but active ultrarunning scene, but most I did not know. There were not many of us, around 30 – mainly British, but a couple of French and Australians too.

Having spent some time together travelling there, we have become a band of brothers. More join us at base camp – Peruvians, looking relaxed and happy. And in that moment I was too. This is what I love doing.

So there it was, the start line. And what lay between us and the finish line was 155 miles, thousands of feet of elevation, a variety of geography, and mildly worrying but exotic and exciting wildlife. This was a new environment for me and one that, if I am honest, I had not really considered as a place to visit, let alone run in. The views at the start of the race from the cloud forest were sweeping and vast. We were high up so could see for what seemed like hundreds of miles. The cloud cover had broken up in the sunlight and as far as we could see land, we saw trees. Mountains and trees.

In Day 1 alone we were going to run through five separate ecosystems. It is so biologically rich and diverse that animals which do not normally coexist can be found within a few kilometres of each other. In short, being there was a privilege.

The race started and off we went. Deceptively, the course started off on a downhill dirt road. Despite the fact we were weighed down somewhat by our full rucksacks, we all set out too quickly, as is customary in a race. After a couple of miles, we turned off the road and finally entered the jungle.

It was a swift wake-up call. The humidity was close and fierce, and almost immediately I realised there was just so much to fall over. These were steep descents breathing in thin air with a variety of trip hazards, some visible and some less so: roots, vines, mud and leaf puddles so deep you could not be sure what you were dipping your foot into. I had been rather blasé about this race and my approach to training for it had been on the mild side. It turns out that running around the Surrey Hills in springtime is not quite enough to prepare you for the thick jungle and sticky heat of the Amazon Rainforest. Not for the first time during a race I marvelled at my own ability to be so unprepared. This was naivety bordering on stupidity.

Within about three hours, my feelings amplified, it occurred to me that I had made a grave error of judgement and that this might turn out to be not the environment for me. Forget Type 2 fun, this might not be any type of fun. I had never before regretted a race, let alone regretted it a mere three hours into one scheduled to last five days.

I was a veteran of hot races and multistages, but I had completely underestimated so many things. The terrain was savage. I do not use this term lightly. It was nigh-on impossible even to walk sections, let alone run them. As the course had been cut into the jungle just several days before, we were among the first people to traverse these routes. Sometimes they were just holes cut through the dense foliage, barely big enough for a human to climb through. Plants were not hacked down to the roots, or had regrown a bit so you had to focus constantly, eyes looking down on where you were stepping to avoid treading on a sharp cut stem, or catching your feet in trailing stems. While you were looking down at your feet, branches whipped you in the face or caught your hair and clothes. So many plants were sharp. If a plant made contact, it would do one of five things: whip you, stab you, catch your clothing, make you fall or even poison you.

Our route was marked by bright pink tape, which was reasonably easy to spot as a vivid contrast to the endless greens and browns, but it also meant you had to have your wits about you while moving along. Looking at your feet, looking out for the tape, looking into the jungle to see what the hell was making that noise – you had to concentrate all the time. This made the whole thing even more arduous.

Very quickly the field spread out – at least, as far as I could tell. I didn't see another runner for hours at a time and I had no idea if we were near the front, in the middle of the pack or last. I don't recall many people passing, but I had not started at the front. It didn't really matter anyway. Experience tells me that the first few days of a multistage ultra are not where the race truly happens. That's always in the second half.

This was the first race I had to wear gloves to protect my hands rather than to keep them warm. My £9.99 gloves from Lidl would prove to be one of the best things in my kit. The mud that we were running through somehow managed to be both like glue and yet slippery underfoot. If you were not going downhill, you were going uphill; there seemed to be absolutely no flat bits whatsoever and it was extremely tough-going. Mercifully, on occasion you popped out of the jungle on to a dirt road. This offered a bit of a respite from the focus required just trying to stay upright and moving along at any semblance of pace.

The jungle is deafening. I have no idea how many decibels count as too many, but it's like having something persistently shrieking in your ears, morning, noon and night. Bugs, insects, birds and creatures all came together in a rattling cacophony that made my ears ring and gave me no peace. Eventually it becomes a white noise, and it is only when hearing something which sounds a little bit more piercing, like a cry, that your attention is drawn back, and you notice the sound.

On Day 1 I fell over very hard, landing on my arm. Incredibly, rather than being in a jungle section with its numerous trip hazards, this was on a dirt road section.

Tired and rather shocked at how hard I was finding the race, I can vividly remember spending the rest of that day hoping it was broken. That would mean no more running and I could just cheer on my husband over the next few days, going with the crew. Upon reaching the finish line, however, I was informed by a race medic after a cursory look that it was bruised but not broken. I would live to race another day – *but do I want to?* I usually start a race feeling eager for more. I was already feeling defeated.

Later Kris, the race director, told me that Day 1 is not really the jungle proper; they set the race up to start with a relatively soft stage so they can see how runners respond to the environment and assess their ability. It is a small taster and test of what is to come. It's the shortest stage and has the least amount of trail.

Fortunately for me, I was not alone. My husband and I had agreed to run the whole thing together. Having company in difficult moments can provide its own comfort – and with that comes power.

We arrived back at camp together for the first night in the middle of the race pack. Some people were still out there enjoying the rigours of the course, while others had made it through faster. This meant we did not have the opportunity to choose the plum spots for hanging our hammocks, but equally, these were not the worst ones, which sat on the edge of the camp and were more exposed. Rain threatened overnight and the camp had a tribe of monkeys nearby. Kris advised us to keep things tethered down and secure. It would have been a disaster to lose any precious food or kit so early on in the race. Anything lost into the jungle night could not be replaced.

We could hear the monkeys howling and screaming at each other in the trees, but it was hard to tell proximity and numbers. I did not want to be on the outskirts of the group. For only the second time in my life, I hung up a hammock.

The first time had been the week before on a practice run in my local woods, to the general bemusement of passing dog walkers. I had borrowed my hammock from the legendary ultrarunner Mimi Anderson. It's the sort that is made for the Amazon, extremely lightweight and it packs compact and small. Once it's hung up, you zip yourself in, like pulling together the skin of a peeled banana. Inside is netting to stop anything within a certain size range from biting. Mosquitos cannot get through, but some ants manage and it definitely won't stop jaguars.

Mimi is an incredible, record-breaking ultrarunner. She's done all the races that require any grit and when I asked her about the Jungle Ultra she said simply, 'That's a toughie . . .'

I should have known.

I was delighted when she lent me her hammock: the thought of being in the very same hammock used by Mimi Anderson had reassured me somehow. I thought that I would zip myself in each night and overnight recharge off her glow, emerging refreshed like a butterfly from a chrysalis, ready to race. The reality turned out differently: every single morning I cursed and swore at the thing, calling it an abomination and insult to comfort.

In truth, my difficulties involved a severe case of user error. Somehow I never managed to achieve a hang that was good enough to give a taut and supportive night's sleep. On the first night, exacerbated by my tossing and turning as I tried to find a shape that would let me relax enough to sleep, the tethers holding me up loosened. My knots were not good enough, the hammock softening and sliding down. By the morning I was

V-shaped, my forehead about 60 cm away from and level with my knees, and my bum touching the jungle floor. The moisture had wicked up, capillary style, through the hammock – and now my hammock, my sleeping bag and the only set of clothes I had and was wearing were soaking wet from the bum cheeks up.

I would have four more nights to try to figure out how to hang my hammock better.

••••

Day 2 was more of the same. Running down a section of dirt road, I saw something spanning the entire track. *A fallen branch? Would a fallen branch be so uniform and straight?* As I got nearer, I could see a regular pattern. *Is that . . . snakeskin?*

It was indeed. In front of me, blocking my progress, was a snake so thick and long it lay across the entire dirt road. I had no idea which end was the head and which was the tail because both ends were hidden by bushes. There was nothing to do but leap over it – and then I did a relatively fast half mile to get right away. Another time I went through a spider's web so thick I wondered if I might have actually bounced off it Scooby-Doo style. I didn't stop to look for spiders, fearing that if I saw how big they were I would not be able to get the image out of my mind and my already bad night's sleep would be filled with spidery nightmares.

I have a real fear of spiders; they genuinely terrify me. I know I said as much earlier, but it's a phobia – and one so strong that when I came home from work one day to find a huge spider in my front room, I immediately left my house and stood outside in the street. After a while a group of school kids passed by and I offered them cold, hard cash to remove the beast. I simply could not step back into the building while it remained.

So yes, spiders were my number-one concern about running in a jungle. The distance and heat hadn't bothered me so much; the prospect of being so near so many arachnids did. Now here I was, surrounded by God knows what, in Peru.

How did I manage?

The truth is, I simply chose not to think. I can be quite good at shutting the door on something and choosing to believe that it is simply . . . not . . . happening. So in my head there were no spiders at all – and when that assumption was pierced by solid evidence in the shape of that huge spider's web, I simply ran away. Handy in a race.

Waking each morning in the cocoon of my back-crunching hammock, I gingerly opened one eye, hoping not to see the silhouette of a spider or any creepy-crawly on the other side of the fabric. On more than one occasion I yelled over to Shaun, zipped into his own hammock next to me, and asked him to get out and check and double-check that there were no spiders on the outside and that it was safe for me to unzip and emerge. Poor sod.

Putting up with my spider-based histrionics, however, paled into insignificance compared to what Day 3 had in store. Looking back, I'm grateful I didn't realise how close to death he was – and am forever thankful to the medics who brought him back from the edge.

The race started off much like the previous two days. For me that meant a sense of dread about what the day held in terms of the terrain, discussions about the length of the stage and a stodgy rehydrated breakfast. The good news was that by Day 3 our packs were getting lighter and today the sun was shining. So, warmer.

My husband, unlike myself, is not one to share suffering. It's just how he operates. Which can be both good and bad, depending on how you look at it. He had been feeling unwell the whole previous night, but had not said anything.

We had set off for more dirt road and even more jungle trails. We were warmer, but what was most noticeable was the increased humidity. It was 100% by Day 3. I had genuinely not realised that humidity goes up that high, thinking that 100% humidity means it's raining. Turns out that there can be rain and 100% humidity at the same time. Imagine being soaked to the skin while also getting wet from the rain.

Humidity can be hard for a non-acclimatised body to deal with. In a dry climate, any sweat – the thing your body releases to help keep you cool – evaporates or can be wiped away. In humidity you wipe it away and more moisture covers you quickly. Your body starts to lose the ability to keep cool – and then you can lose control of your core temperature. At that point, things can unravel fast. You can train for humidity coupled with heat, but in addition some people are just predisposed to be able to cope with it better. I am.

The jungle is not a good place to start losing your ability to keep cool and a jungle a couple of days of hard travel from a hospital is a terrible place. And right then, unbeknown to me, this was happening to my husband; he was now slowly cooking from the inside.

He is usually a quiet person and not one to make a fuss, so maybe I should have noticed when he said his head was hurting and he was feeling a little unstable. Having seen how he was in the Sahara, I thought this must have been playing on his mind and I reassured him that it wasn't that hot. We had got to Checkpoint 2 and I was feeling quite good. Once this day was done, we had only two more. Today's finish line would be over halfway in terms of hours, so mentally this was reassuring.

He surprised me by saying, 'I'll have a little stop and rest here; I'll catch you up.'

I said I would stay, but he refused and said he wouldn't be long. Just minutes behind. Off I trotted, expecting him, as the faster and stronger runner, to be able to catch me with relative ease. After about 20 minutes I slowed, wondering how long he would be. By 30 minutes I had stopped and toyed with the unthinkable in an ultramarathon: going back on the route to meet him. By 45 minutes I had realised that he might have taken a bit more of a rest and was either not going to catch me or not planning to catch me. A little depressed at the thought of finishing this stage alone, I was sure he would want me to press on rather than wait: *we'll see each other at the end.*

Meanwhile, back at Checkpoint 2, Shaun had descended rapidly into a severe and worrying state of heat stroke – a medical emergency. If you are not stabilised quickly, you will die. It's the next level up from heat exhaustion, something we realised later Shaun had been battling while running through the first hours of the day.

From the time he stopped, everything went south. He was complaining of being cold and shivering, a sign of how far his body was struggling to function. He was disorientated and started vomiting.

The checkpoint was manned by medics and they did what they could with what they had to stabilise him.

Meanwhile, I was making my way steadfastly to the finish line, completely unaware.

Eventually I made it to the end of the stage. The first thing I said to Kris King when I crossed the line was 'Can you tell me where Shaun is?' By this I meant could Kris look at the tracker and see where he was on the course.

One look at Kris, though, and I knew something was wrong.

Still vomiting, but at least more stable and in the excellent care of the Exile Medics (qualified medics with a penchant for adventure, who volunteer to assist in these races), Shaun was still at the checkpoint. This would not be an easy extraction, so the decision was made that the medics would stay to see the last of the runners through the checkpoint and then take Shaun back to base camp for further medical help. The only way out was a slow and difficult walk of 3.5 miles through the thick humid vegetation to the nearest road to get collected by a vehicle. Kat Ganly, the doctor taking care of Shaun, kept a keen eye on him as he wobbled and weaved his way extremely slowly through the trees and vines to relative safety.

I waited very nervously at the finish line for the next few hours. Finally, we saw their vehicle bouncing around the corner in the rutted mud road. He was taken out of the car and put on a series of IVs.

This seemed to set him on the road to recovery: he finally stopped dry heaving, napped and eventually managed to eat some Hula Hoops. Crisis averted.

Shaun cannot really remember much about this whole episode, but Kris and Kat do and we are thankful to them both; thankful for their clear and calm communication. Kat also happens to be an astoundingly talented ultrarunner and I came across her several years later at another event. She asked after Shaun.

'You saved his life!' I said.

She nodded, in a matter-of-fact way. She's a doctor; it's what doctors do.

Luckily, Shaun had listened to his body rather than his wife and stopped when he did. If – and only if – he had made it to the next checkpoint, that would have meant a trek of 13 miles out of the jungle to the nearest road. If that had happened, there would have been a strong possibility that the only thing that would have saved his life would have been the most extreme extraction method: scrambling a helicopter from Cusco.

Trying to sleep that night was difficult. Shaun was safe, that was good. But I was exhausted and, zipped up awkwardly in my sagging hammock banana cocoon, it dawned on me: *I am hating this*. The only thing making it bearable was not doing this alone.

Now I'm on my own.

I toyed with the idea of chucking it in too: *it's only running after all*.

Was it worth it? In a single day, it had turned into a joyless and shocking experience. And yet, this was the Amazon Rainforest, that most epic of places. This was once-in-a-lifetime stuff. We had both come all this way and together we had achieved so much to reach this point – *should we both now leave empty-handed?*

How many people can say they have survived five days running self-sufficient through the Amazon Rainforest? Only a handful.

I wanted to be one of them, wanting it more than I wanted to stop. And I really, really wanted to stop.

There were only two days left. The two longest days, the two toughest days – the two days when, according to the race staff, the race comes alive.

I made the firm decision as I went to sleep that it was all or nothing from this point on. *Game on.*

••••

Day 4 stated with a biblical deluge. The start was delayed due to a strong and heavy rainstorm. Huge booming bolts of lightning slashed the sky. The rain might as well have been buckets of water being thrown from the sky. The route was carefully checked, with hardy race staff sent out to assess some of the more difficult parts. Some were rerouted, causing more delays. There was even talk that the course might be cut short. Despite my determination to continue, I prayed for this. With each minute that passed, my keenness to finish this race waned more. Shaun was still in bits, but doing his best to be encouraging, bless him.

This was our holiday, for God's sake. Who does this for a holiday? Well, without going into too much detail there were a couple of very interesting characters in our group. One knew a lot about guns and another was in the SAS. This is what members of the SAS do for fun, apparently. Both of them were the quiet type, not too forthcoming with personal details, and both looked like they could be quite handy in a hostage situation. Nice guys and both were great runners. By the third night SAS Guy, presumably understanding that I'd had a rough day watching my husband return in a crew vehicle, walked over to my saggy hammock, took it down and rehung it correctly. 'I actually can't stand looking at it like that,' he said as he walked off.

Hung up correctly, the hammock was a revelation. It actually passed as comfortable and supported me well for a better night's sleep. I really hoped he would do it again another night, but he didn't and I didn't ask. It's accepted that you are on your own in these events and one kind gesture and the gift of some sleep was more than enough on a very bad day.

Now, that morning, there I was in the pouring rain, aching all over and bitten into a rash. By that point I was eating my food, ants and all, without even bothering to try to remove them. This cavalier attitude to insect eating had started by Day 3. Bugs are everywhere and most of the time you do try to get them off and out and away. But mid-race, you are tired, and you simply get lazier and care less. I can remember looking down at some sweets that were wet from river water and seeing the insect holes going in through the wrappers. I gave it about two seconds' thought and ate them. Those sweets were all I had to eat for that day and one rule of self-sufficient racing is that you don't start dipping into the next day's food, no matter how hungry you get. Start doing that and you will be in dire straits by the end of the race.

So, I looked at the sweets and told myself that my body needed the calories and, hey, here was the added bonus of extra protein. Things get wild on multistage races. Much more quickly than in any other environment, you numb and normalise to things. Next year perhaps we should just go to Spain and sit on a beach and drink cocktails.

••••

River crossings varied in enjoyment from fun to harrowing. Most were done on foot, on your own steam and using your own judgement on the best route to take through the water. The fun crossings were over deep rivers and they were fun because they were the only points in the race when you were not relying on your own energy. On one crossing I was put in a large rubber ring and dragged by a rope attached to a boat rowed by race staff. Battling with the strong current, they ferried over one or two race participants at a time. It was bumpy as we were washed around by the choppy water, swinging about left and right in the current behind the tugboat. We got wet, but we were already wet from the humidity. People pay for this sort of fun on Mediterranean holidays without the jeopardy of falling out and seeing a caiman swim in your direction.

Another memorable crossing was at height, not something I tend to get on too well with, and it was such a thrill and relief to not have to figure out how to cross the river myself. Runners were grouped together in threes and fours and placed in something that looked suspiciously like an old pallet which had been fashioned into seats. We were harnessed in and given safety helmets of sizes more or less appropriate for the size of our heads. Our seats dangled off a zip wire, which was positioned high above a raging river. Two people operated the mechanism to get us across the river relatively smoothly. It was like travelling in the most basic of cable cars and just so nice to sit down even briefly; I almost enjoyed the view!

••••

Day 4 was the first to be tackled on my own. Finally, we were off. I just wanted this race done and out of my life as soon as possible. Although not so long at around 20 miles, this stage was the toughest in term of rainforest terrain. The whole stage is right in the thick of it, featuring two huge climbs and slippery, sharp descents. I spent the day chasing and trying my very best to stay with the two lead female runners. Fuelled by a furious determination and a fear of being totally alone, I didn't want to let these two out of my sight. Both runners were far stronger than me. One, in particular, Kristina Schou Madsen, a professional ultrarunner, is notable for her fearsome attacking approach to events. One of her mottos is 'But did you die?' I didn't know this at the time and did everything within my power and strength to keep up with her.

The thing about the jungle is you really cannot see that far ahead. Someone could be only 40 metres ahead or behind and you would not know, so thick is the vegetation and so twisting is the course. Eventually the women pulled away from me; I simply was not fast or agile enough on my feet to be able to keep the pace. I was left feeling alone and isolated.

The rain had made the already clogged mud even more sticky. The dampness rose up like a cloud and the whole area had a vivid, earthy smell. Vines and roots, woven together, made the entire rainforest floor beneath my feet uneven with every single step. The going was the toughest I had ever experienced. It was on the last climb that I fell hard and slid back down. Lying there like an upturned beetle, I pondered how I had got here. *This is it*, my inner voice said. This was the end. I couldn't go any further.

In races when you decide that you no longer want to be part of the event, you can take off your race bib and hand it to the nearest race official. It's a way to symbolise you are out. The problem with deciding I wanted out at this moment was that there was no race official close by. The next time I would see anyone would be at the finish line, and the previous checkpoint was miles back. There was nothing for it but to keep going forward. *This is what I will do*, I vowed, *and after today I will stop.*

I was hating every single second of my existence by this point. Hating being there, hating being constantly wet and hating the jungle, absolutely sick and tired of the relentless screeching and stupid, endless, shitty climbs. There was simply no other option for me but to go forward, so that I could retire, get the hell out and find a hotel. Preferably with Wi-Fi, hot food and an impeccably well-stocked minibar. That was a very strong motivation to get up and get going again.

I trudged on. Somewhere on this miserably slow progress towards the finish line I saw something remarkable, so unexpected, it stopped me dead in my tracks. The jungle foliage had broken up to reveal a valley. And there, nestled in the valley, I saw something I had not seen for days. Buildings.

It seemed unreal. It looked like a tiny town. There was a large metal building, there were chimneys puffing out smoke, vehicles, dwellings, lights! Electricity! *Could that even be a shop? Oh my god! Imagine if there's a hotel with Wi-Fi and hot food!* I stared for a solid couple of minutes trying to process this. My tired brain and eyes were slowly soaking in the scene in front of me. It was only within that moment that it occurred to me I had not seen anything vaguely like this since arriving at

Manú National Park. Seeing something like that after days of being deep in a jungle blew my mind. It did not look big, more of a village than anything, but emerging from the wilderness it looked like an oasis. This was Pilcopata. The last stop, the last shop, the last place the road goes to before 600 miles of uninterrupted wilderness.

I was near to the finish line. I could have cried. I went into runner mode and ran as fast as my legs would carry me.

Shaun clapped me in. Once over the line I announced to both Shaun and Kris, *I'm done. Out. Absolutely no way am I doing the next day. It's double the mileage, with 6 miles up a river. Nope.*

Forget it.

Not happening.

I don't care about finishing. I can't do it. I'm done.

••••

Day 5. I cried at the start line. I cried with a mixture of exhaustion and fear. This was it, the last time I had to go into battle with the rainforest. It was the day everyone has been dreading; the day we had been building up to.

Collectively we looked utterly disgusting. We must have smelled even worse, bedraggled and stained by the week. Clothes were torn in places, pretty much everyone had cuts on them, everyone had been bitten by something or other, and apparently someone had a case of trench foot.

Earlier in the week, someone had stepped out of a hammock, carelessly barefoot, and was bitten on the foot by a bullet ant. I had never seen anyone hit the deck so fast in agony. It was like they had been shot. It turned out that those critters score the highest on the global pain index of stings. I refused to take my trainers off anywhere near the ground after that.

Now, after a week's worth of terrible sleep in hammocks, of being wet, of limited food eaten out of a bag, I was exhausted. Utterly. I had not changed my clothes or washed all week, because that involved extra effort. I had barely any energy and had no idea how much weight I had lost – at a guess, over half a stone. I could see my ribs. We had already climbed up more than 10,000 feet, and then made countless knee-crushing descents and crossed so many rivers. The climate was hotter the lower we went.

All of this combined to make the last day a battle of attrition. After returning the previous day, I had been cajoled into eating my noodle dinner and getting into my hammock, my desire to stop met with sympathetic nods and gentle words of encouragement.

'So close now!'

'Just one more day!'

'Imagine the beer at the finish line when you are done!'

Kris had given me a pep talk. 'Your experiences with running up to now,' he explained, 'have been with people clapping you; you have run with people around you. Here in the jungle there is none of that. I could tell from Day 1 it was a struggle for you. You can do it.'

Today was to be our last start line. The route was double the distance of any previous day, and featured the longest river section and the steepest climb – 3000 feet straight up in less than 3 miles of mud. We were to run one large loop out into the forest, through some fields, and then along a river back into Pilcopata.

Incredibly there was only a handful of dropouts. We had battled our way this far and most of us now decided that this was exactly what we had come for. We were at the point in a race that we simply had to keep going. We had come so far, gone through too much, achieved so much. The cuts, bites, falls all had to be for something. They could not be for nothing.

This was the last day. We were standing shoulder to shoulder at that start line, a group with a silent and steely determination. *It's us versus the jungle for one last time.*

I swallowed my crying and dried my tears. I made up my mind: *today is the day I do everything within my power to see this race done. Absolutely no way are we going home as a couple without*

*a medal. Shaun wants this. Nothing is going to stop me. Fuck you,
Jungle, I'll show you.*

••••

It had still been dark when we made our way to the start. All the
locals had lined the streets, cheering and clapping as we headed
out. They opened their front doors and banged their pots and
pans. Shouted good wishes. Whistled encouragement.

After the previous few days, this injection of life was utterly
joyful. What must they have thought of us given how we looked
(and stank)?

At that start line I genuinely had no idea how I would do
it – and all these years later, I still don't know how I did. Hours
of that day are lost to my memory, shut out by my brain. My
head went to a place it had never been before, a kind of mental
shutdown not experienced before or since.

There are only a couple of things I can remember. The rest
is gone.

I can remember a bit of the river section. It started around
22 miles in and involved wading up a river for around six miles.
I had made a mistake and not crossed over earlier on, staying
near the bank. With each step I took, I was trying not to lose my
footing on the slippery wet rock underfoot. The water rushed
over my knees, refreshing and cool, but just staying upright was
extremely hard work. After a while, rushing cold water starts to
make your muscles go rigid.

Sometime into this, I realised that the little pink wayfinding
tape was on the other side of the river, and turning away
on to a trail I had missed the best crossing opportunity and
would now have to make my way across to stay on course. The
thought of retracing my steps at this stage was horrible. The
quickest resolution was to swim. Swimming with a rucksack
on your back after 22 miles and fewer than 400 calories for
the day is a challenge. I'm not a great swimmer and got swept
away for several hundred metres. I don't even remember being

frightened in this moment, just that I was trying my hardest to get to the other side. I had no control of myself in the current and I was flapping around, trying to read the water. Somehow, I managed to get to a part of the river shallow enough to be able to stand again and from there I made my way to the bank. Clinging on to plants on the side of the river, I had to make my way back upstream. I did this by gripping on to more plants on the bank and, in the worst parts, dragging myself through the current.

By then I was numb. Numb from the wet, numb from the effort, numb from everything. Vast sections of the day were so numbingly similar to the others, it is hard to distinguish them in my memory.

The other memory I have of this day is one which turned out to be entirely unlike what I had anticipated.

All I can remember is running – through mud and thick bushes, along dirt roads. Wading in rivers. Keeping going. At one point I was aware that it was actually quite dark. I stopped and put on my head torch. Fumbling around to put it on, I was not even thinking about race distance, looking at my watch, or even trying to work out how far I was into the day. All I was doing was functioning and moving forward. I literally had no other thoughts left in my head. *Just keep moving forwards.*

I continued, focusing only on the circle of light from my head torch bobbing around in front of me on the dirt road. After a few minutes I noticed another light. It seemed to be coming towards me.

'Susie! It's just around the corner!'

It was Shaun, waiting for me.

'You've done it! It's here!'

I just stared at him. *Can this really be it? After the most difficult week of my life, can this really be the end?*

We ran into the little town of Pilcopata together. *This is the moment, the one I have been dreaming of all week, the one that I have fantasied about reaching, the very thing that means the end is right in front of me.*

I thought there would be relief, satisfaction, maybe even a tear or sky punch of celebration.

I felt nothing.

Someone handed me a bottle of beer. I tried to muster up a smile for the camera. Nothing. Every last drop of energy, of feeling, was gone. Left out there in the jungle. I was done. It was done.

••••

It's remarkable how quickly you recover from these things. How you can go from utter exhaustion to OK so quickly. Not necessarily muscle-wise (my legs took weeks to recover), but overall physically. Shaun had sourced a simple shack room with a bed in it. No more hammock! He had purchased some crackers and tins of tuna. I ate the food and drank the beer. My first food that had not been drenched by a river or rehydrated with bugs in it. It was, and still is, one of the best meals I have ever eaten in my life. That night, finally able to lie flat and not in some spine-bending crunch, I slept like the dead.

The next day, to the soundtrack of the occasionally out-of-tune but incredibly endearing Pilcopata School Band, the race team and runners assembled for some food and reminiscing about surviving the jungle. The wobbly fiesta music was the backdrop to more glorious food and drinks. The school band had been practising for weeks, bless them. It was musically awful, yet charming, and no one wanted it any other way.

The party was for runners and all the crew. We shared stories of climbing mud, of close shaves with snakes, of struggle, of the sheer extraordinary brutal beauty of the place. This wasn't just the runners telling their stories, either. The medical team who made up the checkpoint staff had their own extreme circumstances to navigate. The team for the halfway checkpoint on Day 4 had set out the previous day to get there and set it up. This had been an expedition of their own, carrying water, medical supplies, communication radios and battery packs, and trekking for 24 hours to set up the station for our safety. Starting out in a truck, they drove up a river for several hours, then took to a boat. Finally, they disembarked to trek for several more hours to set up camp overnight and be in place for the first checkpoint.

As a runner, you care only about yourself and become incredibly self-absorbed. To hear these stories here brought home how extraordinary this event is – and how indebted the runners are.

There are a couple of hazy photos of me at the end and I am utterly dead behind the eyes.

Kris says a lot of runners are a little bit out of it at the finish. He has seen it a lot. 'Everyone is exhausted. It was like you had PTSD. You were blank. It takes a while to sink in.'

In a small field of women, I had managed to place third and I was delighted.

We all journeyed back to Cusco, to hotels with hot showers and white sheets and pizzas.

There, it finally began to sink in. Overall the feeling was one of relief. For Shaun and for me. We all went out and partied hard to celebrate the end.

I learned a lot in that jungle. About staying focused to help maintain resilience. About how much tougher you can be when you simply have to be. About how it is not advisable to go out drinking with a load of medics who have been stuck in a jungle for a week.

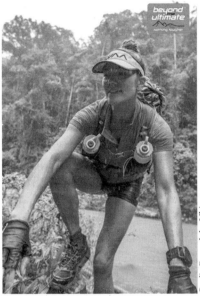

Credit: Beyond the Ultimate

One of 70 river crossings.

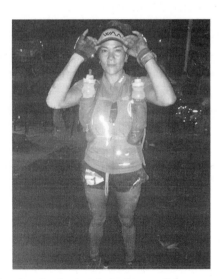

After five days in the jungle and one of the most difficult
weeks of my life, I emerged into civilisation.

7

24 HOURS RUNNING AROUND A TRACK

Tooting Bec Athletics Track, 2018

'The dogs were sitting on the back seat, not very impressed; this was the worst walkies ever.'

'But . . . why?'

I admit it, out of all the things I've done, this one is the hardest to explain.

I have not looked at the weather forecast and frankly that was a good thing. Ignorance is bliss. Ultramarathons tend to be run on picturesque routes or on well-trodden historic trails, leading the runner mile after mile to a finish line a set distance away. Checkpoints can help break up the miles and provide structure and something to aim for on your journey. Sometimes races can be large loops in the countryside, maybe even an out-and-back route, taking in the same course but giving you the opportunity to look at it from a differing viewpoint. This is one of the huge attractions of the ultra scene; new experiences, new places, new faces.

I have found myself in places I would have never seen were it not for running. This is one of the simple pleasures of racing. Ever-changing scenery as you make your progress in a race: hills, views, mountains, jungles, seascapes, deserts, rivers.

Somewhere, you can find an ultramarathon that will show you Earth's wonders.

I am standing in a car park in Tooting Bec, about five miles south of central London. Ahead of me is an unremarkable 400-metre track and a small brick building with a toilet block. A wonder of the world it is not. Skies are grey and light drizzle splatters from the skies, making the whole thing appear even more drab and underwhelming.

I walk over to the track, stepping right to the edge without placing one foot on it. Yep, that's a 400-metre track. Like any other 400-metre track anywhere in the world. The lines divide it up into the standard athletic proportions: 100 m, 200 m, markings for the 1500 m, staggered distances, and a start and finish line. The lane numbers 1 to 8, counting outwards to the edge.

This is my race course for the next 24 hours, this 400-metre loop and nowhere else. This is track racing at its most extreme but the scene is anything but extreme; it is so very pedestrian, so very ordinary that it's almost forgettable, a sight you can see on any drizzly sports field in any regular British town.

Despite the lacklustre setting, the atmosphere is most convivial.

People have arrived and set themselves up for a whole day's racing. Cars are allowed at certain points around the track and they have pulled in to bag various spots, parking up for the next day. Shaun and I are one of the last to show up and opt for the top left turn, just after the corner straightens itself out for the home straight to the finish line. It is one of the few spots left and benefits from absolutely no shelter from any tree. Other pitches are snuggled into corners, under branches. The rain picks up.

Shaun parks up and stays sat in the car while I step out into the rain shower to see what's what.

••••

There are not many of these long-form track races, especially in the UK. This one in particular has a more than a whiff of old school, underground ultrarunning. It forms part of the Sri Chinmoy race series, which are legendary in the ultrarunning scene.

The races are named after Sri Chinmoy, an Indian spiritual leader credited as one of the key players in bringing the practice of meditation to the Western world. Having set up a meditation centre in New York in the mid-1960s, he went on to global influence and success with his messages of peace, calm and focus. Google him and you get a succession of images showing him meeting high-profile people: Diana, Princess of Wales; the Pope; Mikhail Gorbachev. He was a popular fella. He also liked running and was a huge advocate of fitness in general, becoming a weightlifter later in life. It was off the back of this heady mix of belief and fitness that his races, sports teams and running clubs evolved. By the late 1970s there were long-distance swim teams, cycle teams and ultrarunning teams.

Several races now bear his name. This one, to give it its full title, is the Sri Chinmoy Self-Transcendence 24 Hour Track Race.

The original concept that inspired this race is to run so much you achieve a higher state of consciousness. In several Sri Chinmoy races, this elevation of the mind is aided by the fact that there is virtually nothing else to stimulate you. They are deliberately designed for you to empty your mind. A fair few of his races tend to be loops – many, many loops. The longest Sri Chinmoy Self-Transcendence race is 3100 miles around one block in New York. It is officially the longest race in the world, and runners cover the same half mile loop over and over and over again until they stop, become too mentally befuddled, are injured or complete the distance. They have 52 days for the feat, which equates to 5649 loops and is just shy of 60 miles a day. Winners get a T-shirt. By comparison, this 24-hour track race in Tooting Bec is a fun run.

••••

With the rise in popularity of ultrarunning in the past few years, we have seen some quirky and deliberately tedious and testing events starting to crop up. I've seen races around a car park, back and forth over the same bridge, in and out of the same short tunnel. There seems to be some allure in making races ever more boring. The more miserable and repetitive, the better. Whether it's bragging rights or the triumph over the monotony of the challenge or both, this type of race seems to be becoming slightly more popular within the community.

This particular track race was not just about bragging rights, though. At this race elite runners were trying to qualify for the GB Ultra Team. Selection for that made you part of a very small and elite group who had the golden opportunity to represent Great Britain at the IAU (International Association of Ultrarunners) 24 Hour World Championships.

Others were here to run far and fast enough to be selected as part of Team GB for the Spartathlon in Greece. In this infamous race, you run 153 miles and complete the event by kissing the feet of the Leonidas statue at the finish line in Sparta.

Tooting Bec is the same as any other 400-metre track in the world – there is not a lot of space and the field is limited to a maximum of 48 runners. You request an entry from the selection team, and then hope and wait until you get the email telling you you are in.

For these reasons the field tends to be a glorious mix of hardy, experienced speedy ultrarunners, up-and-coming runners who show promise, some well-known faces in the small but vibrant ultrarunning community, and a few who just want to give it a go and see what happens. I was firmly in the latter category.

I did not have lofty goals. It was all about how far I could run in the time. By then, I had run 100-mile races, so the notion of continued running for an entire day was not completely novel, but I had no idea what running in a large circle would do to both my body and mind. There really was only one way to find out.

When I stepped out of the car, perhaps the most immediately obvious thing to strike me was that we were clearly absolute amateurs. I had decided to turn up last, not wanting to spend any more time at the track than necessary. I am not a fan of hanging around at the start of races. In the UK it is generally cold and being at the start hours beforehand serves only to elongate things and draw them out more. You just get nervous and have to ponder what you are about to tackle. So, as usual, I chose oblivion, just trying not to think about it.

By contrast, everyone else was setting themselves up nicely for the next 24 hours. Each runner had someone to feed, water and care for them. Several had multiple people to crew them. They were busy now putting up gazebos, getting heaters out, pitching large four-berth tents. We saw camper vans, minivans, barbecues, stoves; some people even had motor homes and all the cushioned, dry, warm comfort they had to offer. Very slick, professional, considered.

We had rocked up in a small BMW hatchback with three carrier bags of food in the boot. I thought I was being fancy by packing a camping chair for Shaun. We had also brought our two dogs, Roy and Peggy, thinking it would be quite nice for them to scamper around and get some fresh air. The most we had by way of coverage from the elements other than the inside of the car was a small tent for them; a pop-up tent, designed to keep babies covered from the sun on the beach, and so small that a grown human could barely fit their torso in the front flap.

Why, oh why, have I not read up more about preparing for this race? What must we look like to everyone else? I saw a few nods in our direction, even the occasional smiling, sympathetic wince at our set-up. All I had thought I needed was just enough to keep me fuelled until the next day. Ultimately the shortcomings of my set-up would affect Shaun more badly than me. What he would endure over the next 24 hours would prove to be more testing, more soul-destroying for him than it was me.

••••

The race set-up is a well-oiled machine. It has stayed pretty much in the same format since 1989 (it now takes place in Battersea), and is organised by Run and Become, a local running shop inspired by the philosophy of Sri Chinmoy. The premise is as simple as it gets: you have 24 hours to run as many 400-metre loops as possible. Results are ranked by those who have run the furthest distance. However, you need to be out on the track for a minimum of 21 hours for your result to count. Those who stay out running for the entirety of the 24 hours get a notable mention. If you stop running shy of 21 hours, you are classed as a DNF – Did Not Finish.

At the marking for the 100-metre finish line there was a huge gazebo, protecting a row of desks from the elements. Within this, seated behind the desks, were a dedicated bunch of Run and Become race volunteers who each had their own runners to mark, and each time these runners passed by they counted the lap. What a hypnotic task it must be, sitting there counting people running past, especially in the dark of the night. Watching runners filing past again and again requires a certain skill to stay focused. These volunteers rotated throughout the event, sitting for a few hours at a time before swapping out and taking a rest. (Reassuringly, there was in addition a race timing mat capturing distance each time you ran over it.)

Just past this gazebo at the top end of the track, before the 200-metre turn unbent itself out along the back straight, sat another large gazebo. More trestle tables were set up, each with large catering servers. This was the food station, where hot food would be dished up at three set times over the race for all involved, and a bonus hot meal would be served at the end.

Bar the delivery of hot food, the most exciting thing that happens in this race is that every four hours you get to change direction! Anticlockwise running switches at a certain point on the track to clockwise. For six times in the next day, you are rewarded with a whole lap of being able to see the faces of your fellow runners rather than the backs of their heads.

The switch of direction is not there to give you a different view of your competitors, though; that's just a pleasant bonus. It is there to save your left leg from taking the hundreds of incoming track turns. This, as I was to find out, becomes excruciating over time.

••••

I got back in the car, having registered for the race. I pinned my number on my shorts, and Shaun and I gazed out of the window at the series of tents and camper vans all set up as the rain fell on the windscreen. The car wipers scraped in a noisy rubbery drag across the window, clearing the view momentarily, before the rain splattered upon it again, slightly blurring the scene. The dogs were sitting on the back seat, not very impressed; this was the worst walkies ever.

Not a single living thing in that car liked being out in the rain. No one said anything. The windows fogged up. This was about as drab as UK weather got. *Hmm. Maybe it will stop raining soon? That would be best for all of us, really. Shaun doesn't even have an umbrella.*

Mercifully, there was not much time to dwell on our situation. *Well, not for me anyway; the race is about to start!* Everyone taking part lined up, huddling together like penguins against the weather. We were dressed in a variety of rain jackets and head coverings, and wished each other luck. There was always an air of joviality at the start of races — nerves, excitement and an acceptance of what was about to happen.

I placed myself about three-quarters of the way back in the group, which felt about right. There were some extremely talented runners at the front and I knew full well that they would be aiming for a mileage and speed I could not even contemplate.

I knew that the course record for this race was a staggering 166 miles, set by Donald Ritchie in 1991; the women's record was 147 miles set by Therese Falk in 2017. These numbers boggled my mind. I quietly mentally set myself my customary goal of 100 miles in 24 hours.

The klaxon sounded. It was midday on Saturday, 22 September. The klaxon would sound again at noon on Sunday, 23 September. *Off we go!*

As expected, the front runners headed out at a fair clip. My plan was to be slow and steady at the start, and just keep going like that for as long as possible. It was a simple plan, but strangely difficult to execute. I tend to use the contours of a race course to help me pace myself, slowing to a walk on hills and picking up pace downhill. That's impossible on a perfectly flat surface.

Being on a track also triggered a mild Pavlovian response, encouraging me to run at speed. I had only ever run like the clappers on a track, chasing seconds off standard track distances. I knew to within a couple of seconds the time when I should be hitting the 200 metres mark.

Ultramarathon race starts tend to have a quicker first mile before everyone settles down. Here, we had nothing but our own talent to separate us, and the pack immediately fractured and spread out. The elites at the front bounded out ahead, while some people started off in a walk. I tried to settle into the pace of a 10-minute mile, and was lapped before I reach 500 metres. This was the first of countless times I was lapped.

I had already decided to try to avoid looking at anything apart from the track itself, my feet and about five metres in front of my feet, in an attempt to try to savour every possible sight and not burn them all in the first lap. So I was trying very hard not to fixate on any one thing each lap, like a lamp post, a parked car or the timing mat. I wanted to avoid getting into the habit of counting the amount of times I passed it or using it as some sort of benchmark. That, I assumed, would be the very thing that mentally unravelled you each time you stepped over it or ran past it, just by exacerbating the repetitive nature of the event.

Don't look up, I told myself, *give yourself something visually to look forward to. Then in time, you can take in something new.*

That, at least, was the idea, but as I ran around and around the same bit of track just 1 metre wide, it quickly became ridiculous. In minutes I realised its futility. The track was the track.

Now I drank it all in with my eyes as I navigated around. Timing mat, building, gazebo, tent, Shaun, car. Timing mat, building, gazebo, tent, Shaun, car. People wandered in and out of view, ebbing and flowing, crewing their runners. Instead of trying to avoid the view for as long as possible, I tried to notice something new each time: the way a tree branch was shooting outwards at odds with the overall growth of the tree; the shapes within buildings, the triangles, the rectangles. *Where does that fence end?*

The rain continued to fall and around and around we went.

After a while, things synched into a rhythm. People had settled into their paces, and any start-line nerves had been burned off. Just by the timing mat was a huge leader board showing the top 20 runners. I was not on it, going round slowly and steadily at the back with the last eight. I focused on reaching the four-hour turnaround, the nearest thing to a checkpoint, giving us all something to look forward to, a well-earned benchmark for progress through the day. Yup, I was actually excited about changing direction.

••••

Every single lap at the top corner, Shaun asked me if I wanted anything. In a flash of crewing genius, we had come up with the plan to bring a tray, on which to place all the usual suspects for race nutrition. The word *nutrition* was used loosely here. The tray had things like crisps, fruit, crackers, a pot of rice pudding; a standard checkpoint condensed on to one tray.

Shaun stood like a wonderful ultra-butler each time I came around, offering up the tray of food. Invariably the thing I quite fancied in that moment was not on it. I asked for something specific and he took the tray away and rummaged in the carrier bags in the boot of the car. And it was always there on the next lap.

Even if I requested nothing from the tray, the timings of each lap were such that he did not have much time to put the tray away, shut the boot and get back in the car, because as soon as he did, he had only a couple of minutes before he had to get out and top up or tweak the tray and come to meet me. Each of my laps was, however, a long enough period of time to get fairly rained upon. It was for Shaun a painful no man's land of back and forth between the boot of the car and me. I was covering the same 400 metres over and over; he was covering the same 10 metres over and over.

After several hours of this, I realised how hideous it must be. He is not the sort to complain and even less so when crewing. I tried to help by saying: 'Give me four laps!' so that he would at least be able to grab a few minutes sitting in a car seat rather than standing up and being rained on. The dogs were having none of it in, snoozing in the car. Shaun called a friend to come and collect them.

••••

It was time for the first direction change — which was nothing short of thrilling. At 4 p.m., exactly four hours after the starting klaxon, a cone was placed on the track at a strategically calculated point. We all ran up to and around the cone going into the middle track lanes for one lap only. Faces! Smiles and high fives! *How jolly we all are! Look at us all running this silly race in this weather! Good to see you! Fancy meeting you here!*

Then, after that one lap, it was exactly the same as the previous four hours, just in the opposite direction. I was not entirely sure that I was expecting anything less, but I tried to take in this new perspective with fresh eyes. Tried to take in and notice new things around me for a while, only to find, after just a few laps, that running anticlockwise is as mundane as running clockwise.

Time passed: around and around and around we all ran, and the rain continued to fall. Sometimes it lightened to a drizzle, and then returned to rain again. Shaun stood on the same corner, offering up his little silver tray of food. The delights on offer would occasionally swap. A slice of orange perhaps? Maybe you want to try some salt and vinegar squares? Babybel?

By the next direction change, back to clockwise, the evening was drawing in. At this point, I had been running for eight hours and felt reasonable, but was so grateful for the change in direction.

Rather like a checkpoint, changing direction became something to count down to mentally: it divided the race, broke down the 24 hours and, of course, provided a fleeting moment of interaction. It was also welcome as running in a large circle really, *really* made one leg ache. A large proportion of the track was taken in a bend, which began to take its toll on muscles and joints. The first few hours on fresh legs, this was not really that noticeable. However, as time passed and the muscles started to fatigue, the ache from the repetitive running action crept in.

This pain was exacerbated by two things. At Tooting Bec, the first problem lay right underneath us and there was nothing we could do about it. Most athletic tracks are made from a synthetic rubber, and good tracks are created with a product called Mondotrack, the crème de la crème of track surfaces. All top-end sports events are run on nothing less. A synthetic track provides grip, a slight bounce and cushioning underfoot. This is brilliant for preventing injuries and gives the athlete a tiny bit of energy back. The track at Tooting was not made of anything vaguely cushioning. It was made of concrete – unforgiving. Not something that seemed a problem for the first few hours, but several hours in it was feeling very tough on the tootsies. My feet were starting to ache, particularly my left foot. This was not my first long race to take up to or over a day, but my experience until now had been on trails with their mud, grass and roads, the mixed surfaces providing Nature's own Mondotrack for your feet.

The second thing that exacerbated the ache in this race was the reality of being left to your own thoughts for so very long. With nothing new to see at all, your mind wanders until it latches on to a thought and then you are stuck with it going round and round your mind until the next one drifts in. I generally try to distract myself from what is happening within my own body in ultramarathons. I try very hard to avoid focusing on any twinges or niggles that invariably happen when you run for so long. Having changing scenery helps, as you can look about you and fill your mind with: *I wonder how old that house is? Is that the sea on the horizon?* and other mundane but mildly entertaining thoughts. I prefer not to have earphones in a race, sometimes saving it as something to look forward to. At times in a long race the music can turn into white noise and you end up back in your own head anyway, with your own thoughts.

On the track, with not a huge amount of stimulation visually, it was hard not to think about the pain in your feet and the increasing rigidity of the leg running on the inside of the track. You really were just left alone with all the thoughts in your own head. It was like being in a non-stop living daydream.

Sri Chinmoy had called this the Self-Transcendence race for a reason. His theory was that you can expand your mind in monotonous situations, as you realise that you and your mind are much more than your surroundings: *expand one's self-consciousness to conquer the mind's perceived limitation* is the logic, apparently.

At only eight hours in, and with a mind that kept returning to how much my feet were bloody hurting, I wasn't there yet.

Runners had settled in and found their own groove. The elites up front were lapping me and lapping me again, ticking off miles at an astonishing rate. I studied their running: their pace looked like they were running a fast marathon, striding out confidently but comfortably. It dawned on me that they were indeed running fast marathons. Running around this track faster than my own personal best.

It was not really the sort of race that you buddy up on and pass a few miles chatting with a fellow runner for a bit. I am not really sure why it was this way; perhaps it was because most people there were seasoned ultrarunners, confident within themselves and knowing how to handle being alone and running for so long. Maybe it was because they had a specific time goal as their focus. Or maybe it was simply that if you were next to someone chatting, then you were by definition in Lane 2 – and running a small extra distance every lap which would not count. Unthinkable, frankly.

My friend Sophie Raworth came along to witness the race, incorporating it into her long run of the day. She turned up early in the day too, hood up against the drizzle, giving me some words of encouragement, chatting to race staff and crew, cheering – and promising to return with some hot chips for me later in the evening. Eating hot chips had been an excellent strategy in a three-day, 130-mile race around Anglesey. On the late afternoon of the second day, which was a reasonably gruelling 63 miles, I ran through a small town along the Menai Strait and spotted a chip shop. Not having much race food to sustain me over the three days, I made a spur-of-the-moment decision and ran into it mid-race. Looking and smelling very much like I had run a double marathon, I ordered some chips to take away: 'Don't wrap them, extra salt please!'

Holding on to the hot paper package in one hand, wooden chip fork in the other hand, I ate them jogging along. It proved to be exactly what my body needed and I managed to rally for the final tough, hilly night section.

Here at Tooting, as the rain became heavier and the temperature gently dropped by a couple of degrees, I became fixated with the arrival of my hot chips. Every 400 metres I asked Shaun for an update on when Sophie and the hot chips would arrive.

I do not even recall being that hungry, but there was a comfort in the smell and taste of chips, and everyone knows that eating chips just makes everything better.

Will they arrive soon?

Perhaps I can have a little sit-down and eat the chips!

What a little treat that will be, a sit-down in the camping chair, resting my aching feet with my hot chips! The package warming my hands, the smell of the vinegar wafting up and piercing my nostrils while my tastebuds tingle with the salt.

It's just what I need, the food that will make me feel all cosy and fuzzy on the inside! Hot chips! Are they coming soon?

They were not. Sophie was not returning with chips. Something had come up and she had to look after her children. Shaun broke the news gently. I was devastated. More devastated than you ever need to be about fried potatoes.

For some reason, small things can upset you much more in ultramarathons: your emotions run higher as you become tired and you are liable to be triggered by minute things. A laughably emotional overreaction about the lack of chips proved a low point for me. I knew that I would never be able to reach Sri Chinmoy self-transcendence if I was going to obsess about salty junk food. I had to move on.

I was offered a jacket potato from the food tent. I did not want it. A jacket potato is simply not hot chips.

••••

Dusk had closed in around us, the streetlights were flickering on, the orange glow highlighting the raindrops still falling against a darkening sky. Same track, same sights, same loop, same weather. I passed the leader board, where the names at the top were clocking up huge mileage, 60, 70 miles. My plodding meant my name was still not even gracing the top 40 runners; I was still in the bottom eight, doing my own thing. We were so close together as a group on this tiny bit of land in South London, and yet we were all running our own races, chasing our own personal goals. The only thing that changed was the daylight into night, and the volunteers in the tent counting us around.

I was doing my best to acknowledge them on most laps and saying a few words when I could. Focusing especially on the volunteer whose job it was to count me specifically as I went past. This was partly because I wanted to acknowledge what a job they had, counting people running past a soggy gazebo for hours on end, and partly because a small part of me wanted to be sure every lap was ticked off.

They waved back at me, nodded, raised a hand. It must have been quite exhausting for them too. Focusing so you don't miss a runner, in not very warm and rainy conditions which made everything more challenging mentally. When they swapped over, they let you know: 'I'm off for a break now! This is your new lap counter!'

Somewhere around 11 p.m., in my increasingly tired state, I decided to call a ultrarunner I knew to ask him a ridiculous question.

I pulled my phone out and dialled up Robbie Britton, veteran of this very race. I had met Robbie years ago. By 'met', I mean I had seen him flying around ultra courses in the UK. In the early 2010s, he was one of a small handful of names on the scene, along with

James Elson of Centurion Running, who were really blazing a trail for the rest of us to follow at a more leisurely pace in the next decade.

I have no idea what part of my brain decided it would be a good idea to consult Robbie, but in the last few hours I had needed to stop for quite a few wees – more than usual – and I thought Robbie would be able to lend some sage advice. He had given me solid advice on the odd occasion over the years.

The phone rang.

'Hello? Susie?'

'Hi, Robbie. Weird question, but how many pisses are too many? I have had loads in the last three hours.'

'Do you feel fine?'

'Generally speaking, yes.'

'As long as you are hydrating, then it's fine.'

Some more small talk, then: 'Thanks!' and I hung up.

It was only several loops of the track later that I remembered that Robbie lives in France. I had called him out of the blue at midnight his time, asking about my pee rates, like he's some sort of a medical expert. Poor guy, but what a top bloke for answering the phone and trying to make me feel better.

••••

We were closing in on midnight. Halfway. Shaun was being an absolute trooper in the rain. He must have been utterly miserable, watching me move in a soggy jog around and around, throwing mild hissy fits about the lack of chips. The convivial atmosphere had become more subdued. While Shaun stayed awake in the rain, crew members were taking it in turns to nap, or watch over their runner. No such luxury for my crew.

The track quietened down and there were just the sounds of the runners' trainers slapping the watery, rock-hard track as they made their circular progression, around and around again. The rain kept falling, softer now, creating drizzly misty halos around the floodlights and black night sky. It became a curiously peaceful space with the rhythmic sounds of footsteps and raindrops and quiet conversational murmurs of those awake.

This was a night-time state of calm and a state of running that had become almost meditative. *Is this where the magical self-transcendence occurs?*

••••

What sounded like a rusty trumpet tunelessly pierced the night sky. Noisy voices approached the track. Laughing and whooping and tambourine rattles. What on earth was this breaking the methodical serenity?

My friends.

With the grace and aplomb of a hen party in full swing, Charlotte, Emma and Sarah burst forth from the gates yelling: 'Oi, Oi! Keep running! One more loop! Looking good!' followed by another raspy blow from a dented wheezy trumpet.

'Chan! I found this!' Sarah bellowed at me across the track, waving the trumpet. She was wearing a bright pink feather boa over her Dry Robe jacket. Emma had a tutu on over her clothes. Charlotte was dancing to absolutely no music like Bez from the Happy Mondays.

These three are my running buddies. We have known each other for years and spent hours – and still do spend hours – pounding the trails of Surrey and Hampshire, each of us with our own individual and often different running goals, but all of us drawn together by our love for running. Each one has their own accolades to their name and all have run ultramarathons, so they were well aware of how hard it can be. Sarah in particular is a very talented runner; running competitively since she was a teenager, she wins races on a regular basis such is her strength and experience. Humble but focused, she wins anything from 5Ks to 100Ks and is consistently fast. A regular open water swimmer too, she has a sign on her van which reads 'All Dry Robe and no knickers'.

On countless occasions we have all propped each other up during races and reassured each other during tough training runs, egging each other on around tracks and goading each other across tough cross-country races.

We met at our local running club and perhaps we ended up being drawn to each other because we never took the science of running seriously. We just loved running and kept it simple. If we had been inclined, we could really have got down to the nitty-gritty of minute miles and making sure we did our warm-up drills correctly and all the other bits that go with serious training blocks, but we never really got too involved in all that. We just turned up to run and train together, and there was a time where we all ran pretty well for our clubs. Sarah was always out in the front. Emma and I were around the same speed until it got to a long distance; as soon as it went to marathon, she had the edge on me. Charlotte was pure power; her sweet spot was short distance. I had to make do with trying to keep her in sight in anything 5K or under.

We had bonded over running, but over the years grown closer as friends. None of us are particularly girlie or huggy people, but we show our friendship through an unspoken sisterhood of support in whatever our running journey and life has thrown at us over the years. The misery of injuries, the agony of near-miss PBs, the tired and testing days when being a mother is difficult, the days when work is getting on top of you. We knew between us we had made a safe space, talking freely in training runs, or bouncing stupid WhatsApp messages into the group, sharing gossip and memes, and whinging about things knowing there would be no judgement. These are my people – and here they were, utterly ruining the tranquillity.

••••

In any other situation, I would have found their arrival absolutely hilarious. Twelve hours deep into a race of 100 miles, I would have liked nothing more than my friends to show up blowing into a trumpet and trying to get even a single note out of it, and hurling terrible insults at me just to make me laugh. The sight of them dancing around to their own jokes dressed half for winter and half for a carnival was pretty funny, but I really wasn't sure if it was going down well with my fellow runners or those crew trying to sleep. In all honesty, the noise of them after hours of steady quiet crewing and running was grating.

I shushed them quiet as they made their way over. At the sight of them, Shaun handed over his tray and sat in the car, locking his door. He needed a well-earned rest off his feet and something waterproof and warm. Plus he was reacting like he always does when we all get together – he gets the hell out of there.

Sarah surveyed the scene. Her expert runner's eyes narrowed, analysing the small mob of us shuffling, jogging and running around a track in the dark of night and pouring rain. 'Well, this looks shit. How you doing?'

I was not in a great place. My left foot hurt and I still had not eaten hot food. I was starting to struggle to eat and this was in turn making me feel tired. Yet the presence of my incongruous friends had buoyed my mood and awakened me. Not wanting to let them know that it was, in fact, as shit as it looked, I rallied a little bit. I'd had no idea they were going to show up, especially so far into the race, so it was a surprise, a kind surprise. They had deliberately come at this time of night knowing there would not be much support on the track. They ran alongside for a few metres each lap, giving me pep talks and generally being quite nice, rather than going straight in with insults – which made me think I must have looked like I was struggling. I was grateful, so very grateful. They left after about an hour, heading quietly back into the night and leaving me once again with my own thoughts. So I decided to think about them and their kind gesture: travelling through the night to get to South London, giving Shaun a bit of a break and all the things they had cobbled together to create a little carnival party for me trackside had warmed me. Thinking about this for some time after, I picked up my pace.

I settled into a rhythm again. Charlotte had made me eat some baby food pouches, which had gone down very well, and I was feeling a bit better. Peace and quiet restored, the darkness of the night seemed to be so close around us. Beyond the floodlights illuminating our narrow track was silence and blackness.

••••

It must have been around 2 or 3 a.m. and I was tired. My body was tired and I was so very tired of all the thoughts in my head. Bored of my inner monologue, my head had gone through all the usual conversations and concerns. Thoughts had one by one slipped away. My chin dropped a little and my gaze softened, my sight not really focusing on anything in particular but a general area just ahead of my trainers. The white lines of the tracks stood out against the wet dark lanes. At times the lines themselves looked like they were floating ever so slightly above the track, hovering and bending in their own dream-like suspension against the puddles. My eyes were not taking in the track in sharp focus; everything was faintly drifting. My feet instinctively knew what was happening and stepped out one after the other, after the other. The rain continued to fall from the gloomy sky. I was so wet and I had been out in the rain for so long by this point it was not even registering against my skin. My brain was drifting into a state that bordered on sleeping while running. There was nothing but running . . . running . . .

I stayed in this state for an unknown time. It's all rather blurry, but after a few hours I became aware of a familiar kind and gentle voice: 'Hello, Susie, I've taken over from Shaun for a bit.'

It was Tim Jones, another person from the running scene, who had turned into a very good friend over trail runs and race meetups. Tim is universally acknowledged by everyone who knows him as one of the nicest people on the planet. What I like about Tim is that he is indeed incredibly kind and thoughtful and generous, but you can swear your head off or make an inappropriate joke and he will find all of it terribly funny. He is a very pure soul and up for a laugh too.

And now he was standing in the exact spot where Shaun had been for the previous 16 hours, bar the one-hour break provided by the midnight hen party.

Such was my night-time fatigue by this point that it took me a couple of laps to cement the idea in my head that he was, in fact, here. A couple of laps to react. Shaun was nowhere to be seen, having almost immediately taken himself back into the car in an attempt to dry off and rest. It must have been quite the welcome for Tim.

Each time I came around, he asked what I needed and offered up various goodies on the slippery silver tray, just as instructed. He was crewing with a fresh zeal that had, unsurprisingly, ebbed away in Shaun as he slowly froze in the rain. Exhausted from standing, fetching, offering, placating and watching me run nowhere in circles, he had run out of dry clothes, he was hungry and he just needed a break. No other runner had come with just one crew member.

And Tim had come to the rescue. Setting an alarm for 2.30 a.m., he had driven through the night from his West Sussex home to Tooting. He really is a top friend, but in my exhausted state I was barely able to communicate.

Apparently, any time I passed him by, I mumbled about hot chips, lamenting my loss like the death of a family pet. Tim went over to get me some leftover food from the race tent and returned with half a jacket potato cut up. I had point-blank refused this earlier when offered it by Shaun, but doing that to Tim felt really rude, so I took it and tried to eat while still walking around. The jacket potato had taken on a strange woollen texture. Knowing that food always helps in ultramarathons, I kept trying to get it inside my mouth, cutting bits into smaller and smaller chunks. The rain was catching in the polystyrene container holding the potato and turning the chopped-up bits into potato sludge. I managed to eat the watery mix, though, getting in vital calories.

At this point, I was trying my best to put on a brave face even though my feet were now seemingly on fire, from the heels all the way to the balls of my feet. Each step hitting the track delivered a thud of pain to my tender soles. The rain started to get stronger and heavier, and after so long it really was starting to get challenging. 'Just one hour without rain, please!' I heard someone cry.

The long, dark, cold, wet night proved to be too much for some and people were dropping out. After around 17 hours from the start, I noticed my name finally gracing the leader board! At some point overnight I had crept into the top 40 out of 48.

••••

Dawn. The heavens opened. It was that thick, heavy, lashing rain that is like turning on a tap. The sort you know will not last long, but which will, if you get caught in it, ensure you get soaked. The rain now found ways to seep down my neck, little cold drips of it trickling between layers and filtering down on to the skin of my back and chest. It crept upwards somehow into my trainers until I could only feel wet socks squeezing between my toes. Tim had acquired an umbrella from somewhere and was watching me, doing his best to be encouraging with facial expressions and hand gestures. The normal rain had been bad enough, but at around 19 hours in, this seemed unnecessarily cruel. My foot was really hurting. *This race is so stupid.* I wanted to have a little cry, but not in front of Tim.

Shaun had reappeared, though, so I called him over and started to cry, saying I hated it. The heavy rain washed the tears off immediately, so it just looked like I was whimpering.

'You are close now. Just one more four-hour turnaround and you are done!'

The darkness changed to gloom and then finally the daylight came, lighting up the scene in the closing hours. In the cold light of day but in heavy rain, we looked even more bleak. All the merriment and bonhomie had evaporated. Some people disappeared off the track, taking refuge in the warmth of their vans and tents for short breaks when the rain was at its worst.

A hardy few stayed out on the track – myself included, because I was fearful that if I got inside the car I would never be able to get out, to open the door back into the rain, into the cold, into a run. Sitting down in the car would be game over.

I treated myself to one break: saying I needed the loo, I went into the toilet block, sat down on the ice-cold loo seat, lid down, and rested my head against the loo roll like a pillow. I gave myself a luxurious five minutes out of the rain, sitting like a saturated stray having a micro nap. Five minutes only. Any longer and it might have been impossible to get going again.

Some people never emerged from their tents and vans. My name edged up a few more places on the leader board, but I was feeling dreadful by this point. Empty, in pain and, despite trying so very hard to believe otherwise, 20 hours of being in the rain had destroyed my soul. I was sick of it.

Then, just when I thought conditions could not get any worse, a lady with a piccolo turned up, playing a jaunty tune at our end of the track. Bless her for trying to cheer us up, but it went on and on. Sharp, shrill notes seemingly in no particular order, boring into your tired head every time you went past. At the far side of the track you could still hear it, and the whistling came in and out in volume as you moved around the track. This was torture. Even Tim, the nicest man on the planet, was finding it excruciating. Nobody said a word. But I wanted to take her stupid piccolo and hurl it as far away as possible.

We made the last turnaround. Just four more hours to go and I was reduced to a shuffle. The race director was watching me from afar.

••••

I had no dry clothes left and now, in the final four hours, a sequence of events was about to unfold which no one watching the race in that moment could have predicted.

I had weathered the storm, literally, and now all I had to do (so I thought) was to keep moving round. I was sick of it, but no way was I going to stop now and have all that work be for nothing. No way.

The race director came over to chat to us. He had some news.

'You need to layer up or get changed into something warmer, or I'll have to stop you. I'm worried you may be getting too cold. Some runners are struggling and have retired, and I don't want you to get hypothermic.'

He was looking after me diligently. Admittedly my shuffle and miserable face were probably telling a story of suffering. *But can't I keep going?*

I became aware that I was shivering.

I argued that I felt fine despite how I looked. He was kind but firm: layer up against the elements or get off the track and into the warm. Those were my options. Now we were in a pickle. Neither Shaun nor Tim nor I had any spare dry clothes. Everything was soaking wet. I had only what I was wearing by this point: shorts and T-shirt and a thin jacket. Any spare tops were soaking wet and drying in the car. I changed my trainers to a spare pair we found in the boot, hoping this action might appease the race director. It was not enough.

This cannot be how it ends, surely!

Then someone standing near us waved Shaun over. I had not noticed her as part of the small morning crowd. I watched them chatting to Shaun and then, incredibly, right at the side of the track in the pouring rain, she started to get undressed. She stepped out of her waterproof trousers and unzipped her hooded jacket, revealing underneath a set of normal clothes.

'It's OK, I have a coat! I'll go inside for a bit!' she hollered as I got nearer to where she was standing. This kind bystander had watched what was unfolding and realised that my race was in peril. A total stranger had taken off their own clothes, and got herself wet and cold on my behalf to save my race.

The warmth almost immediately made me feel better. My numb muscles started to warm, the waterproof clothes doing their job against the rain. I began to feel less rigid and my gait became less strained, more normal, and I started to move better.

I did not want to let this kind woman down, so I started to make the most of being warm and got running again. It did not feel so bad!

At 21 hours there was a sudden drop in runners. This was the minimum race time you could get to and not register as a DNF. People I had seen running disappeared off track and later emerged with fluffy hoodies on, drinking hot chocolates under covers. My name went up some more places on the leader board.

Then, like a blonde vision appearing through the rain, came Sophie. She had returned! I was so pleased to see her. Even better, she had not arrived empty-handed.

'I felt so bad about the chips! Have this!'

She handed me a coffee cup. I barely drink coffee, but it was warm and she had come all this way to bring it to me. I necked the drink in four satisfying gulps. It was so sugary, it tasted delicious.

Turned out, it was seven espressos with five sugars.

Like rocket fuel.

Warmed up, happier and caffeinated off my tits, I felt a wave of energy sweep over me. More people had gathered in the rain to watch the closing stages of the race, friends and family turning up to cheer those of us left on the track. Cat Simpson, a friend and a Team GB ultrarunner, came along with McDonald's Hash Browns for me. I ate as much as I could.

As I picked up my pace, the small crowd started to cheer for me each time I passed by. I responded with a smile, a wave and, feeling more boisterous, the occasional air punch. I was closing in on my goal of 100 miles and suddenly loving running again.

Something happens to your energy in races when you know you are doing well. You think that you are tired and can go only so far. Then you realise that your race is actually not going so badly and the energy fills your body, lessening the aches and pains. I was feeding off the cheers and started to overtake quite a few people. The race director shouted as I went past, 'It's 18 laps, Susie, and then you make 100 miles!' This endorsement from the very person who had worried earlier about me even finishing gave me even more confidence. It occurred to me too that if he had not insisted on me getting warmer, I might not have been here.

A cursory look at the leader board showed me I was now in 20th place, the fourth-placed woman, and there were 40 minutes left on the clock. The woman in third was just 1 mile ahead of me, which was four laps of the track, and she was walking. *It's all or nothing from this point.* I gritted my teeth and tried my best to stay at a reasonable pace.

Breaking the 100-mile mark brought huge cheers from the small assembled crowd, from the volunteer gazebo, from the race director, and from Tim and Shaun, both relieved to see me finally moving well. I only had eyes for the woman in third. *Can this really happen? Can I podium in this underground, renowned 24-hour track race?* I pushed as hard as I physically could. I lapped her once, twice, three times . . . Then she started to run.

It must have looked like the lamest of races to the finish line. The minutes were counting down and we were both trying to run our best pace. It was still raining and we were both drenched, tired and rigid with the final effort, both of us head down and driving, racing each other for the trophy.

I lapped her again and now it was 11.58 a.m. Now it was all about clinging on for just two more minutes. All of those times I had been to an athletics track and raced, against friends, against Sarah, Emma and Charlotte, I had raced that familiar circuit hard until my lungs burned, my leg muscles felt like acid and my heart felt like it was in my throat. This could not have been slower, but I gave it absolutely everything I had left.

Midday, the race finish klaxon echoed around the track. It was finally over. All runners had to stay exactly where they were when it sounded, so the final distance could be measured accurately. I came third – just. After 24 hours of running around the same loop, there was one single lap in it – 400 metres between the woman in fourth and me.

I had finished next to the woman who won, Sarah, clocking up the most miles. We high-fived each other, both of us bent over and clutching our legs. She had run 30 more miles than me: I ran 103; she ran 133. She is just incredible. The winning man, Michael Stocks, ran 154 miles.

It was finally over. I sat on the puddles in the track for some time. There was the small matter of the trophy ceremony and then we could at last get dry and warm.

When I stood up, my left foot hurt so much. I did not know it at the time, but it would turn out to be my longest-lasting injury, taking nearly seven months to heal fully. Running around that track and changing trainers towards the end had damaged my feet; the trainers were slightly too small and my feet slightly swollen. I had crammed them on, forcing my toes to curl ever so slightly in the shoe for the last few hours. My tendons were so inflamed, the shape of my foot actually changed, the tendons so swollen they had pushed the bones around. Even today, all these years later, my left foot is a different shape to the right one.

I could run short distances for the months that followed, but nothing longer than 4 or 5 miles. I reverted to short, sharp sessions, all of these on a track – I was not quite that sick of it, returning over and over again to get my runner's fix.

••••

After more than a whole day, the rain started to thin out to a light drizzle now that the race was done. I went inside the clubhouse building and was given a new top to wear. I dug out my woolly hat and mercifully, finally, I was able to take the painful trainers off my weary feet, sliding into my flip-flops. I looked very much like I had been running in the rain for 24 hours. Soggy, dishevelled and limping.

Geoff Oliver was pride of place at the awards ceremony. I had seen him out on the track throughout the race. A sprightly 88 years old, he was a veteran of the race, having run it several times previously. He had a steady strategy for staying dry with a variety of impeccably waterproof clothes and a flat cap. He stayed on track, moving in a gentle jog, and covered 77 miles.

He broke no less than eight world records on that day. We were in the presence of greatness.

Within minutes of finishing at midday, he presented himself at the finish ceremony looking extraordinarily dapper in an ironed shirt, tie, perfectly pressed trousers with a crisp crease down the front and polished shoes.

He was already a legend in our circles, but we all marvelled at his post-race admin, which was more on point than the rest of us put together. It took a Herculean effort for me just to take off wet socks, while he had changed and dressed for the occasion. We all clapped heartily as he collected his award. Sophie, more impressed by him than anything else she had seen that day, got him on BBC News.

••••

Shaun and Tim missed the entire ceremony, attending to the car. It turns out if you open and close the boot several hundred times and switch the heating on and off all day, you will completely drain the battery. It was now totally flat. As if they had not endured enough after the longest, wettest day ever, Tim and Shaun now had to jump-start our car so we could finally go home.

On the journey, the sun rays started to seep out from behind the grey clouds.

I clutched my trophy, grinning. 'I loved that!'

Shaun looked at me with a tired smile I had seen so many times before. 'How do you never remember? You hated so much of it! You complained, cried, whinged!'

Maybe I really had reached a state of self-transcendence; I could not recall those bits with any clarity. All I was left with was a huge sense of satisfaction, a very warm feeling from knowing how incredible the running community is, a very sore foot, and, despite being utterly exhausted, the inability to be able to sleep for hours, thanks to the seven espressos.

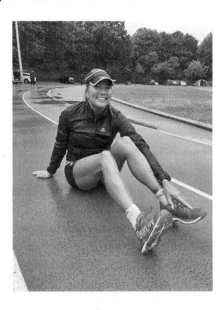

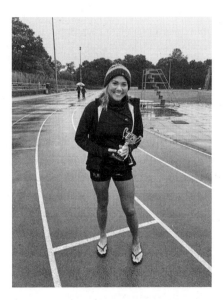

Soggy, dishevelled and limping – but I somehow managed to place
third in this physically and mentally demanding race.

8

GUINNESS WORLD RECORD ATTEMPT, ALL WELCOME

Kingston University, 2016

'Internally I was doing my best to quieten the voices
of doubt and concern which were creeping in.'

It is not every day you realise you can break a world record.

It's 2016 and I am running in the laboratory of the sports scientist Chris Howe. We had met a couple of years earlier. He worked at Kingston University, a venue that formed part of my training for the Marathon des Sables.

Their Sports Science department is well equipped and has, among other things, a heat chamber.

Heat chambers are as grim as they sound. Small spaces which can be controlled and set up in a way to recreate the climate of a hot place, and used to train in. This one looks like a very innocuous small outbuilding on the main campus at Kingston. From the outside it could be a plant room or storage. It has no window and sits about 4 m² with one door. Inside to the left is a work bench for the scientists, on which sit some science bits and bobs (no, I did not excel at chemistry or biology at school), and to the right is a door into another space with a digital display on the outside. There is a small window in this door and in the wall so the scientists can see directly in.

The door is heavy, with one of those huge, pull handles you see on industrial walk-in freezers. Step inside and you are in the heat chamber itself. It is sparse in here with the bare minimum: a treadmill and a rudimentary exercise bike. The floor looks easy to mop. There is also an electric fan, which I vowed never to use, though I always end up asking for it to be switched on. The ceiling houses some industrial gubbins that presumably create and pump out the heat.

The only thing in front of the treadmill is a plain white wall and on that the only thing to look at is a poster, a chart ranging in a rainbow of colours from green to red with some descriptors of how you are feeling. Green is good, red is bad.

Kingston is only about a 30-minute drive from me, and this small and somewhat joyless space became familiar to me as I used it to train for deserts and jungles. I spent hours running and sweating on that treadmill.

The idea is to build up your heat tolerance in the few weeks before your hot climate race. Ideally you leave no more than a day or two between sessions so that your body starts to acclimatise to running in the heat and starts to sweat more quickly to keep you cool. Chris would make it as jolly as could be: loud music was always blaring to keep spirits high and you distracted. Which was necessary because things were pretty much the same each time. You were weighed before running. Chris took some bloods. You went in and started running.

Each day the heat was slowly turned up, slightly more than the previous day. I generally started around 26°C and usually ended up somewhere in the mid 30s running for around an hour each time. When training for the Marathon des Sables, I ran with a weighted pack filled with tins of beans and bottles filled with water, replicating race conditions as best as possible.

The digital display outside the space shows the temperature and also the humidity, which rises in the room the more you sweat into the atmosphere. Chris watches through the window and periodically, with the precision of a sports scientist, puts his gloves on and measures your temperature by way of an ear thermometer, then asks you to point at the green to red chart on the wall to describe how you are feeling.

There are two ways to keep an eye on your body temperature in the heat chamber and this is the less scientific way. The more accurate way is to have a rectal thermometer up your bum for the entire session.

Several notable athletes come to this very heat chamber to train. You have to be quick to get a space as it's the best way to prepare your body and is available for only limited periods of time. We all book on rotation and in the couple of weeks leading up to the start of the Marathon des Sables, Chris spends hours in there monitoring, measuring and pushing us to get stronger in the heat. The legendary Sir Ranulph Fiennes used the space in 2016 when we also ran the event. He opted for the more accurate measuring of body temperature. Usually the athletes fit the device themselves in privacy, but Sir Ranulph, empowered by the extraordinary life he has led, is fazed by precisely nothing. He just dropped his trousers and bent over, so Chris had to do the honours.

I'd put that on my CV if I were a sports scientist.

••••

It's always a gruelling session. It starts off feeling mildly suffocating in the heat, which is always much warmer than training runs in the UK. As you work through your time in there, you may feel tingly and slightly dizzy; heat exhausts you in a way that simple running does not because your body is working hard to keep you cool even as you are running. Afterwards your kit is wringing wet. You twist your clothes and the sweat comes out like they've been dunked in a bathtub.

We are weighed on the way in and out, the measurement converting directly to how much you're sweating out. Each time I lose around 1 kg.

In this heat chamber I trained for each Marathon des Sables and also prepared for the Costa Rican jungle. Over time I got to know Chris well, sometimes making him stay in the heat and chat with me to help pass the minutes, which can really drag when you are working so hard. Chris spent his youth as a top model, strutting his stuff down the catwalks in Paris and appearing in glossy magazines for high-end designers and brands. He also understands ultrarunners, at complete odds with the glamour of his youth. He himself is an extraordinary ultrarunner, having taken part in loads of gnarly races, including the Western States 100 and UTMB (Ultra-Trail du Mont-Blanc), two heavyweights of the ultra circuit. He is achingly modest with it all, and a very genial and calming presence.

••••

Ultrarunning is a relative newcomer to the sports scene and there has not been much research behind performance, and how the body reacts and copes in such extreme environments, and for prolonged periods of time. Chris's PhD examines the science of it all. Part of his research involved gathering data on people as they ran long distances. This obviously needs to be done in a measured way, using the same criteria from one case study to the next. Ultramarathons vary so much; even the same race on the same course can change from one year to the next. Weather plays a huge part in defining the running conditions and affecting the course underfoot.

Having mulled over different ways of being able to take data in a way that would be consistent for various people over the course of a few months, Chris ended up settling on this: participants come to the Sports Science Lab and run 50 miles on a treadmill. They are weighed and various measurements are taken, like bloods and VO_2 (the rate of oxygen your body is able to use during exercise), which are then also taken periodically through the experiment. Mental well-being is monitored too, with runners being asked at regular intervals how they are feeling. Any liquids or food consumed are noted, measured and tracked. The treadmill itself is recording the data. You can run walk, stop and start again, like you do in an ultramarathon. Chris concluded these criteria are the easiest way to ensure that conditions are equal from one person to another, regardless of the day they run.

Unsurprisingly, not too many people volunteered to run 50 miles on a treadmill, but there was enough for Chris to do his research. Without much thought, I volunteered too, as did my husband, and we chose one weekend to get it done. He went for Saturday, I went for Sunday.

At the time I had just finished training for an Ironman. This meant that I had swapped out some of the running for cycling. I'm not the best at cycling, to be honest, and it took me forever to get anything bordering on an adequate training time in the saddle. Unlike ultrarunning, five hours was apparently not enough, especially not at the slow speed that was all that I could manage. In the lead-up to the Ironman, I had decided my time was best spent focusing on swimming, as open-water swimming seemed to trigger my fight or flight response with worrying ease. Generally every time I swam in open water felt very much like a controlled panic. In fact, there were several times I did experience a full-blown panic attack bobbing around in a murky lake and it was terrifying. My friend Charlotte, who ran at the same run club as me, also played water polo for Great Britain. She spent hours helping me gain confidence and working on my stroke. We worked both in the pool and in the lake, and after several weeks of her one-to-one training I was only marginally better. The swim is at the start of an Ironman and, not wanting to fail at the first hurdle, I diligently swam miles every week trying to get better and stronger. By the end of all that training I was, at best, mediocre – which was good enough for me.

At the start of training for the Ironman in 2015, the running continued at the same rate, as I had the small matter of the Marathon des Sables to get out of the way. With all the swimming and running on the go, there was no time for the cycle training, which remained neglected for weeks.

In the end I had around 11 weeks to get bike race fit and that included a two-week taper. So, nine weeks then. *How hard can it be? You're sitting down most of the time!*

I had totally underestimated cycling. Cycling is hard. It turns out that cycling a couple of miles back and forth to work on a fold-up bike is simply not enough to prepare you for 112 miles of Bolton's finest hills. When I practised my first 100-mile bike ride, I took so long that I would have been timed out of Ironman and failed. Spooked, I took part in a 'Sportive', an organised large group cycle ride. But, unfamiliar with the cleat pedals, I fell off the bike at the start line and was so slow that by the time I had made my way to the finish they were deflating the finish line arch.

I did not enjoy the sensation of cycling at speed. I was slow going uphill and forever on the brakes downhill, and it all felt like a chore. Cycling needed more time and work. I didn't have time, so I ended up cycling as much as possible around my full-time museum job. From my house in Farnham, I cycled halfway to London, then hopped on a train towards the city centre, then got off to run into work – and did the whole thing in reverse to get home. I did this multisport commute several times a week. It was one of those times in my life where I look back now and have simply no idea how on earth I managed to do all the training and still continue to be a mother, hold down a job, shop for food and make sure the cat did not die of neglect. True, it left me in a near constant state of hunger and I felt like I had not a single second or ounce of energy spare.

It turns out that cross training, rather than simply running, makes you very strong and fit indeed. Who knew? Propelled by the considerable momentum of these swimming and cycling efforts, I sauntered in to the Sports Science department of Kingston University ready to run 50 miles on a treadmill with virtually no thought in my head about what this would be like.

All the necessary pre-run checks and measurements were taken, and on a table in front of the treadmill were my snacks and drinks, and weighing scales and all sorts of charts for Chris to fill out, as well as equipment for measuring things like my saliva. I did not ask what it was all about, just complied like a good volunteer, doing as directed and getting on the treadmill. Armed with a banging 12-hour playlist, I had absolutely no expectations of time or running performance at all.

I ran. And ran some more. And more. The good thing about treadmills is you can just lock into a pace on the flat. It seemed relatively manageable, so rather than having a break walking up a hill like I might in a race situation, my legs just kept going, and going. There were no checkpoints to stop at and chat, no views for taking photos. About 35 miles in, I realised I was making very good time. My legs did not seem to be affected by the repetitive nature of the treadmill. I decided to dial it up a bit, now giving myself the arbitrary time goal of sub eight hours – faster than I had ever run the distance and seemingly totally manageable.

I hopped off the treadmill, 50 miles down and just shy of eight hours. *Job done.* I felt good! It was one of those days where things seemed to come together. I do not recall any bit that was particularly tough, or boredom, or anything negative at all; the tunes had helped, my legs even felt OK. A positive experience all round and even, dare I say it, fun!

I tweeted about my day on the treadmill, thanked Chris for letting me be part of his research and went home to eat pizza.

Halfway through my fifth slice, scrolling though Twitter, I noticed that one of my friends had tweeted me back. Had I continued running at that pace, they said, I would have broken the female 12 Hour Treadmill Distance World Record. Yes, that is a thing apparently. Not much of a thing, I discovered after a little bit of research, but a thing nonetheless. Treadmill world records seem to be broken down into sex, time and distance. Twelve hours, twenty-four hours, male and female, and so on. Not surprisingly, few people have a go at breaking these particular records and the 12-hour female record was tantalisingly close at just over 60 miles. I had run 50 in eight, which would have given me four hours to knock out another 11 miles. I finished feeling so good and strong that the thought of running another 11 miles seemed almost easy!

I sent Chris a message: 'Ha! Wish I had stayed on now!'

••••

I woke up the next morning still thinking about it. A world record and one for running too! My age played part of the allure. How many people in their forties get the opportunity to break running world records?

What if I tried again, specifically trying to break the world record?

I sent Chris another message: 'Could I break a world record on a treadmill and if so will you help?'

A few weeks later, sitting in a café on the campus, Shaun and I met up over a cup of tea with Chris and Hannah Moir, then Senior Lecturer and about to become Professor at Kingston. Both had come armed with statistics and facts based around my run paces, taken from their numerous readings of me in the heat chamber and during the treadmill experiment. I had come armed with enthusiasm and the vanity of wanting to break a relatively unknown world record.

Surrounded by students tucking in to their jacket potatoes and lattes, we chatted over possibilities. Do any of us have the time for this? And will I even be fast enough? I'm a mid-packer in the ultramarathon.

It did not take too long to decide. I might not be the fastest, but I was certainly keen. We would try to break the world record for furthest distance run by a female on a treadmill in 12 hours.

Game on.

••••

It's one thing deciding you want to break a world record, and another and totally different thing even getting near attempting it. First, you need to find out what is required to validate a world record attempt: unless Guinness is satisfied that all is above board, nothing will get into the record books, so what's the point? There are various stories doing the rounds, making some very questionable claims about long-distance record attempts, so the only way to secure validation is to be Guinness Recognised.

Chris wrote to Guinness saying we were attempting the record and asking what we needed to do to get our attempt verified.

A while later, Guinness wrote back – 23 pages explaining what had to be in place before, during and after the attempt. These included all sorts of details, some of them obvious: for example, the treadmill has to be calibrated and pace verified as correct, independent witnesses are required, the whole thing must be captured on camera, and the recording must be continuous. Some rules seemed less obvious, but with a world record at stake, they seemed reasonable. I was not allowed to touch the handles of the treadmill at all because this could be seen as taking the weight off my feet and cheating. If I needed to go to the loo – highly likely over the course of 12 hours – the treadmill would have to come to a complete stop before I was allowed to step off. Hopping off a second too early with the belt still moving would mean a minor distance untravelled by me.

Then there were things which had not even occurred to us as something to consider. Independent witnesses had to record the distance I was travelling, there had to be at least four at any given time and they had to change every three hours, with none of them repeating the task in the allotted time. They were not to be my friends. The attempt had to take place in a space that was open to the public and advertised as such.

My fun project had turned into a huge task.

We split the workload: me doing the running, Shaun supplying moral support, and Chris and Hannah organising and doing absolutely everything else.

We set a date a few months ahead – January 2016 – to give us time to organise it and to work around the university's term time and our respective lives. To be honest, I did not think about it too much in between deciding it was happening and the target date itself. My regular running training schedule continued, just keeping things ticking over. I did not undertake any specific targeted training for the world record attempt. It had seemed quite attainable based on my previous effort and so, once again in my running life, I made the assumption that everything would be just fine. What I did not take into account is the fact that I would no longer be in the shape of my life from hours and hours of training for the Ironman triathlon in the summer and the Marathon des Sables nine months previously.

A mere week after the treadmill experiment, I cycled Ride 100 – the 100-mile London and Essex event. It was fun, but I was totally over cycling that summer and decided I never wanted to sit on a bike for that long ever again; I put it in the garage. The rest of the year's training was pretty much a matter of me coasting. Lots of easy running, meeting my mates and running on the trails, and no cross training at all. Without even realising it, I was no way near as fit as I had been in the summer. You might think that this would have occurred to me. It did not. As usual, my somewhat laissez-faire attitude, which could get me to the start lines of epic races, could also work against me. Simply, I did not quite consider the enormity of the task ahead.

••••

January arrived. Behind the scenes Chris had been organising on an epic scale. I had not fully appreciated the level of work.

The day before the record attempt, I made a visit to the laboratory to familiarise myself with the set-up.

Chris, with the precision of a scientist, had left no stone unturned. There was signage marking the way from the street to the lab: 'Guinness World Record Attempt, All Welcome' plus an arrow.

It was not a straightforward journey through the campus to the lab: doors were propped open, and tape and cones marked the areas where the public could stand. Guinness wanted the event to be open to the public.

Somewhat less straightforward, the treadmill had been calibrated. A team had flown over specifically to do that and supplied the university with a certificate. Tables and chairs lined one side of the room. On the tables were all the paperwork. Forms to be filled out of distances, names, times, signatures.

A huge display of the distance and pace was rigged up so that people could track how far and fast I was running. A TV had also been set up linked to a camera. It turned out that setting up continuous filming had been a bit of a headache. After various experiments Chris realised that the popular and go-to sporting camera, the GoPro, had the capacity for filming and storing only around five or six hours of footage. Somehow he had to come up with a method of filming and storing footage, and keeping the whole set-up powered, for 12 hours minimum. After testing various possibilities, he set up a YouTube channel to broadcast the whole thing live, saving it on the internet forever.

There was a table for all my race food and drinks, which would have to be handed to me; I would not be able to reach them at all while running.

And right there in the middle of the room was the treadmill. Not just any treadmill but a huge beast. At least twice the size of the standard you see in a gym. It stood nearly a foot off the ground, and the running surface was nearly six and a half feet long. As for the standard display in front of the runner, this one was industrial-sized. Built for experiments. Built for research. Built for endurance.

As for the treadmill on which I had run 50 miles, that was sitting neatly next to the giant treadmill, looking tiny in comparison. It was there for friends to run next to me periodically, to help boost my mood and keep me company.

I took in the scene, took in the huge treadmill, took in all the equipment in the laboratory. It had been set up and organised for days now – and all of a sudden I was not sure if I wanted to run for 12 hours on a treadmill. The whole thing suddenly seemed very real and rather intimidating. The feeling came over me like a wave.

I did not say anything out loud.

In fact, I had said hardly anything to anyone about the event, not really wanting many people to know until the deed was done. My plan was to keep it under the radar. A handful of people knew, close friends and a few from my running club who had offered to come and run next to me. One friend, Sophie

Raworth, did not realise I was keeping it close to my chest and sent out a tweet: 'Tomorrow my friend Susie Chan will try to break a Treadmill World Record!'

Piers Morgan, of all people, retweeted it, calling me mad. People started commenting, tweeting, retweeting.

Word had got out.

This is it, then. After all the work Chris had done, it was out there in the big wide world, and there was only one thing for it: to give it a go – me, an ordinary mum from Surrey and someone who is bang average in races. As much as I wanted to, bottling it because I simply did not fancy it any more was not an option.

One more sleep and I have to attempt to break a world record. For God's sake!

••••

Everything was in place. It was early – we had decided to go from 7 a.m. to 7 p.m. Unbeknown to me, Chris was having huge anxiety about various things that could go wrong – the fire alarm going off, the equipment failing, the independent witnesses not showing up – but he hid his concerns well.

Luckily the witnesses had not actually been too hard to source. A call was put out to the students: *Want to be part of a World Record Attempt? Who wants in?* All they needed to do was sit and watch a woman run on a treadmill for four hours, noting distance and time. Sounds reasonable, but the reality is that after a short period of time it is rather dull and horribly repetitive. All the student volunteers were on a roster, and we had enough doughnuts and fizzy drinks to feed them all for days.

The Volunteer Witness Roster started off strong, with six students turning up before 7 a.m. on a Saturday. Not a single whiff of a hangover, which was one slight relief for Chris and Hannah. I was oblivious to their worries, though, as I was internally battling my own nerves. I engaged the part of my brain that can shut things out and switched on the one that helps me through a lot of my long runs. Call it bravado.

I was full of 'Let's make this happen!' and 'We are going to break a world record!'

You might think there would be a bit of fanfare at the start, but it was all rather humdrum. I stepped on the treadmill, checked and rechecked my bottle placement, tightened my ponytail, and Chris started the treadmill. Due to the size of the thing, there was no control screen, no buttons in front of me; these were all on the side, to be operated by someone else. The machine had been built by the treadmill specialists h/p/cosmos and was so big that Kingston University had made a step up on to it for me.

Seven a.m. and I started running. A few of my friends from my local run club, Farnham Runners, came along to support and run on the smaller treadmill next to me. James Warren was first up, running beside me.

It took me less than two miles to realise I was going to have a very long and challenging day.

••••

Some days when you run, you feel great, like you are flying.

Then there are the days when it all feels normal, no more difficult but no more easy than other days. You are just out there getting it done. I get lots of days like this.

Then there are the days where for no reason at all it is a slog. You can be running at an average pace, not doing anything particularly different, and the running is a chore. It feels harder, your legs feel heavier, like wading through treacle.

This is all part of being a runner. It's par for the course. Except today was not just any training day, my route could not be adapted, there was no option to slow down, or a choice to stop and put my hands on my hips and take a selfie. I had to keep going. Internally I was doing my best to quieten the voices of doubt and concern which were creeping in after only 20 minutes had passed, way too early. I switched up the bravado a notch, chatting away to James, big smiles and waves to people. *Maybe this feeling will pass.* (Sometimes it does on long ultraruns and you settle in.) It did not. Time passed and it did not feel any easier at all.

The speed was set in kilometres rather than miles. Despite all the running in my life, I can still never figure out the conversion from miles per minute to kilometres per minute. Some things are best left ignored; it is what it is, after all. I had specifically requested not to know my minute-per-mile pace and let Chris be in complete control of my speed. He used my performance from the 50 miles to work with and set the parameters.

'Just have it on at the pace I need to be and I'll run it.' One less thing for me to worry about and one more for Chris.

My fastest marathon and 10K had both been run when I was unaware of my pace. I was over a year into running before I got my first GPS watch that told me pace, distance and other stats. At the time these digits meant a lot to me: I used them to mark myself against previous performances, as a benchmark to how well I was doing in my running and overall fitness. Seeing the numbers work in my favour and give me confidence was fantastic. Equally, missing the paces I was chasing brought misery. It would take maturity and time to realise that you simply cannot get faster and faster; it's just not sustainable and, more importantly, most people only really care about how fast they are running, not you. My watch's failure in both the marathon in Abingdon and a 10K around Dorney Lake saw me run faster than I thought possible and brought me personal bests. Sometimes it's just better not to know and worry about how you can keep the pace. This was the state of mind I was hoping for during the next 12 hours.

••••

Friends came and went on the treadmill next to me. Sophie Raworth nearly derailed the whole thing a few hours in by stepping on to the treadmill, unaware that it was turning over at a low speed. Close to falling flat on her face, she reached out and nearly grabbed me. My heart rate spiked, and the incident did not go unnoticed on the livestream.

A succession of Farnham Runners, all supportive and jolly, racked up miles. As did I, under the watchful eye of the student witnesses and Hannah, who was hawklike watching me to ensure no rules were broken, in particular the rule that I could not put my hands down on the side bars. This was relatively easy to avoid because the machine was so huge – until I needed a wee, when the natural thing when stepping off is to reach out for and hold on to a handrail.

The most common question I get asked in relation to this world record is: 'What did you do if you needed a wee?'

Well, it wasn't an ideal situation. For a start, slowing down the treadmill and bringing it to a halt took a little time, and getting it going again after I had stepped back on was not that snappy either, because it was so big it needed several seconds to get up to speed. I had to be really careful not to touch the handrails, and as time went on the process of getting off and on the treadmill slowed a bit, all of which ate into my overall pace.

The next problem was the proximity of the nearest toilet. It was out of the lab, along a corridor, through several doors and up some stairs. Assuming that I would need several loo breaks in the course of the day, we agreed I did not have time for that. So for the next 12 hours I had a bucket.

Some element of decorum was maintained by putting it in the shower cubicle in the next room to the lab, saving valuable travel time and energy going up and down the stairs. I spent the first few hours working my pelvic floor nearly as hard as my legs, trying not to need a wee.

••••

The hours passed. I ran miles and miles. My *fake it till you make it* attitude was working. I had run through more difficult things in the past – difficult terrain, weathers and temperatures – but this was still tough. In different ways. Inevitably this is an event that's tough, both physically and mentally. But there were factors I hadn't considered. When you run outside, even on a track, there will be minor variations and unless you are terribly gifted, your pace will also fluctuate.

Here I was locked in to one pace, each step being exactly the same as the last, over and over and over again. You end up using the same muscles in exactly the same way.

Having my close friends next to me as a distraction helped. If you do anything, anything at all — whether that be running, walking, sitting down, standing, gardening, reading, knitting — for 12 hours straight it becomes hard work purely through boredom. We had all sorts of things on the go to alleviate the tedium. I had curated a varied playlist, which was uplifting and loud, and at times people danced around me, making the atmosphere in the room fun. There were times when the space was buzzing and I fed off the energy.

The students were enjoying being part of this and, incredibly, loads of people came in to watch. They ranged from random people off the street, to people who had somehow heard about it and were driven by curiosity. Hannah recalls that more than a hundred people found their way through the campus to the lab that day. A few friends turned up unexpectedly, which was a lovely surprise.

I was still struggling, but all these things combined certainly made me feel better at various moments. Having so many people invested helped fuel the part of my brain that can drive me to finish lines out of fear — fear of looking weak and fear of being a failure.

A screen had been set up in front of me to show me the Twitter stream. I was very active on the app back then and we had a hashtag — #SusieWRrun — on the go. Things started off quietly, but as the day went on more and more people were jumping on the hashtag and watching along online. The live feed was a fixed camera without sound, because we were unsure about the legality of broadcasting the music playing in the lab. It wasn't riveting viewing; we had set this up as a way to record the whole effort and had not anticipated anyone actually wanting to tune in. Despite this, the stream audience grew and grew. At one point, thousands were watching.

Our hashtag started trending on Twitter. Messages started pouring in from all sorts of people from all over the place. They were on display on the screen ahead of me, generous and kind messages from people wishing me well and willing me on. Paula Radcliffe was tweeting about me. Paula Radcliffe!

People from all walks of life were coming in and talking to me next to the treadmill. This began as a happy distraction and something which was enjoyable. They had come in to find out what it was all about and offer support. As the day wore on, though, the conversations got harder and harder. It was the same sort of questions over and over: 'Why are you doing this?' The short answer is: Because I can. 'How are you feeling?' Increasingly awful. 'What do you do if you need the loo?' There's a bucket.

After about eight hours of this I quietly asked Shaun to act as a buffer, and physically stand between me and the people coming in, answering their questions and chatting on my behalf. I did not want to be rude or ungrateful, but eight hours of intermittent small talk was adding to the mental exhaustion.

Every so often the music would crank up and Charlotte or Shaun would bob around dancing with no self-consciousness at all to lift my spirits. The ups got shorter and shorter and the bravado started to wane. I had managed eight hours reasonably fine, but then suddenly everything dropped off a cliff. It was hard enough to pretend to the people in the room that everything was fine, but I had got to the stage where I did not want to speak to anyone at all. I was waving and smiling in the lab to everyone around, but as soon as I caught Shaun's eye I did my best to convey silently how hideous it was starting to become.

I started to feel a little queasy. It was a specific queasy feeling too. The same sort of nausea that you get from reading a book in a car. This feeling while running was a new experience for me. *What on earth is happening? I've run a lot further than this and been fine.*

Chris worked it out. About three feet in front of the treadmill – and me – was a blank wall and then, slightly to the left, the screen with all the tweets. And that was all I'd had to look at for the last eight hours. 'Your body is detecting motion, but your eyes are not. You are seasick.'

Great.

This was not something that could be resolved, I would have to tough this out. My pace did not drop and I ploughed on, trying every so often to look to my left and my right and to my feet to mix things up a bit. Looking around gave my vision some depth of field. It was tricky because looking to my left or right made me feel unstable, but it did take the edge off the nausea momentarily.

Then, just when I thought that would be the toughest thing I would have to deal with, things took a bit of a turn.

To be perfectly blunt, my stomach had had enough. My guts were not happy – with me, the treadmill or the junk food. More pressingly the seasickness was taking its toll. The next few trips to the bucket were grim. Shaun had to hold me up by the armpits; my quads could not quite handle the squat. There are some moments in your own life which really should not be shared within a marriage. We had been married for only six months, short enough that other couples are still very much in their honeymoon period. It was not our most romantic moment.

••••

There was nothing for it but to try my best from this point onwards. Still on course for the world record, I could not afford the slightest drop in pace. This would mean that the buffer we had planned, the extra distance over the current world record, started to shrink. We had wanted to get to over 70 miles, shooting for 72 or 73 miles. The increasing trips to the bucket and my loss of bravado were all chipping away at my spirits – and pace.

By 10 hours in, I really had to focus very hard on the finish line and getting the job done. My energy was waning and I started to feel most unwell – sick, tired and, by this point, fed up. This was now noticeable to all and everyone in the room started to rally round. We had come too far in the day to fail; it was not an option. All these people had not put in all this work for me to let them down and have it slip away, not in the last two hours.

Somehow I ground them out, those next couple of hours.

Finally we passed the record! Now it was all about clinging on to make it safely past. As soon as I had broken the world record, though, my body had had enough. It was a bit like running past a finish line at a race, having everyone cheer for you and then carrying on just for the sake of it. These extra miles were the toughest ones. The job had been done and now we were in a no man's land of seeing how hard I could push through. I was running on empty and there was nothing for it but to slow to a walk now and again, clawing away at a new record as best I could.

There is no way I am the fastest female runner, nor the strongest, but how do you measure resolve? Determination? At no point did it cross my mind to do anything other than to keep going, to keep moving forward for the full 12 hours. Proud of the fact I did not bale as soon as we broke the record, I managed to bank a few extra miles.

At 11 hours, 59 minutes and 50 seconds, finally it happened: we were in the countdown to the klaxon.

'Ten . . . Nine . . . Eight . . .' Everyone in the room chanted the numbers. 'One! Done!'

I had run 68.5 miles, and felt every single one of them. I lay down on the treadmill clutching my stomach while everyone around me cheered. If I had not been feeling so sick in that moment, I would have joined in.

••••

The aftermath of that moment was a bit of a whirlwind. At some point during the last 10 miles I had been asked if I would like to appear on *BBC Breakfast*.

Sure, why not?

Turned out *BBC Breakfast* was filmed in Manchester.

As I lay there on the treadmill enjoying a moment of stillness, someone handed me a phone. The person at the other end was telling me to be on a train from Euston to Manchester in an hour's time. We did not really have much time to gather ourselves or think. Shaun, Chris, Hannah and I were to get on the train, be put up in a hotel for a few hours, and then be on the *BBC Breakfast* sofa by 6.20 a.m.

In my head for the last few hours had been the tantalising thought of going home and having the biggest, cheesiest takeaway pizza, ice-cold beer and a lovely sleep in my own bed. Not tonight. Tonight was going to be an egg sandwich and bag of crisps on a train to Manchester.

In the lab we popped a bit of champagne (*the stomach won't mind, right?*), had a few sips, thanked everyone, took a cheesy group photo and got ready to go to Euston Station all rather rapidly. Since the original plan had been to head home afterwards, I did not have anything at all with me – no overnight things, nothing to wash with, brush my teeth or hair or anything to wear on TV. Charlotte Hanson showed what a good friend she is: she undressed and gave me the clothes she was wearing, stepping into my absolutely minging run outfit.

That really did cap off a day that showed me just how incredibly supportive and extraordinary the running community is. Friends, family and total strangers had rallied, all gone above and beyond, invested time, energy and encouragement. The end result really was a group effort; the part I played was small.

••••

On reflection, I see now that I did not really realise just how extraordinary that episode of my life was; I was so lucky.

Regretfully, I forgot to apply to be in the *Guinness World Records* book in time, so I did not appear. However, once the record was verified, the certificate was sent to me and hangs in a casual humble brag in the downstairs loo.

I have never seen the *BBC Breakfast* interview and do not ever want to watch it. I have virtually no recollection at all about what was asked or said. Chris was great in the interview despite being sick with nerves. I made for less good TV, as I was so out of it on lack of sleep and general fatigue and, by this point, Imodium.

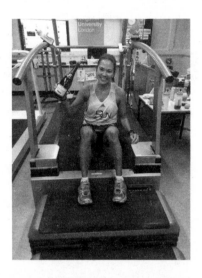

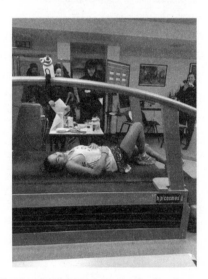

World record broken! Champagne – and a lie-down – to celebrate.

9

SEEING THE SIX STARS

Boston, Berlin, Chicago, London, New York, Tokyo
2014 to 2017

*'The thing about running is there is always
another race.'*

Making the famous Boston start line was by no means easy. My first marathon had been a training approach that was disciplined and structured, followed by a respectable but near-miss time of 4 hours, 5 minutes.

That was Paris 2011 and I can vividly remember trying to cling on to the four-hour pacer, who was running along with balloons tethered to him. I had been ahead of him for a fair distance, when suddenly I was enveloped in a large huddle of runners. I saw his balloons bouncing around in the sky above him and declaring, '4hrs'. I had no idea how far in I was or how my race had been paced as I did not have a watch.

My legs were shot. I felt more broken than in any long training run, yet I tried my hardest to stay with the group. Even so, minute by minute the pacer and his group eased ahead of me until finally I could not see him.

Crossing my first marathon line was agony and bliss in equal measures. Someone said to me that running your first marathon is both the best and worst day of your life, at the same time. So true.

Delighted with finishing, though not wanting even to entertain the notion of running that far ever again, I simply knew I had to go back and try to get under 4 hours. I had been so close to my goal, which infuriated me just enough to try again.

This is how it starts. You try for a time, get it or miss it and then keep pushing. Goal posts shift, aims narrow, targets define themselves further – and the next thing you know, you are running for six days through a desert. At least, that is what happened to me.

I broke 4 hours in my second marathon, and then the quest became sub 3 hours and 30 minutes. This one was even harder, and included one of the toughest and most soul-destroying marathons I have ever done: Edinburgh 2012. The training had not been as structured, but with much more race experience under my belt, and this time with a watch to help me pace myself, I set out on my target minute miles. It all seemed possible when I went through the 17-mile marker. People around me had started to slow, so I clung on to someone in a yellow shirt who seemed to be maintaining his pace, cutting through small pockets of people. Jaw clenched, I was fighting burning quads and ever-tightening calves. I was hurting but maintaining pace. Checking my watch (which I had since invested in), I was closing in on 26 miles and bang on pace to just nip in under 3 hours 30. Then I looked up to see the 26-mile marker in the distance – still a fair way away. It was pure suffering by this point; I put everything I had within me into those last few minutes. My quads felt like they were full of acid burning my muscles to the bone. I suddenly started to feel very dizzy, took off my sunglasses and threw them to one side. In that moment I thought I would rather faint trying than ease up on pace; the agony until now had to be for something. This was all or nothing.

I crossed the line in 3:30:51, having pushed for every single step through gritted teeth for miles.

I sat down immediately after the finish line, just metres past, and remained unable to move for half an hour despite race staff trying to move me out of the way. Broken from the racing, from the effort and from the crushing disappointment, I felt hollow, defeated, crestfallen. It was then I noticed the Edinburgh 2012 medal that had been placed around my neck. It had twisted around and from the back looked exactly like a cock and balls. (I wasn't the only one to notice; it went viral.)

In disappointment there is learning, and it took only a large portion of chips, two large glasses of Shiraz, a stuffed crust pizza and a chat with my friend Emma Passmore, who had run the race too, for me to realise that I had tried my best. There is simply nothing else you can do but try your best. I gave it my all – and my all was 3:30:51.

I went to bed that night accepting my effort and pleased with my marathon progress. After all, I had knocked off over half an hour in under a year.

The thing about running is there is always another race.

I would go on to crack 3:30, which became my goal finish time for a lot of marathons. I went through a period of time with my running when I could just turn up to a marathon and run sub 3 hours 30 mins. It just came to me.

My times improved and, although I was by no means rubbing shoulders with the nippy club runners and elites, I realised that I was not doing too badly for someone who ran for a hobby, and who had taken it up later in life and had only been running for a couple of years. Crucially, it was something that had given me a new lease of life, a new focus, and I was loving it. Boston Marathon became the next goal.

••••

Boston is the oldest marathon in the world and the ambition for thousands of runners, because you need to qualify to make the start line. Qualification standards are on a sliding scale depending on age and reaching the standard does not guarantee entry. Only the fastest are selected.

By this point I was several marathons deep into my running life and considered myself something of a veteran of the distance. I worked hard to get under the qualifying standard and applied. I was accepted. I was off to run Boston!

I had entered the race with my long-lost cousin, Sam. After nearly 40 years of not knowing each other, we had recently connected – and then I discovered she was a fast runner! We aimed for this race together and we were both delighted to go. It was a great way to get to know each other more.

Diary planning has never been my strong point and my Boston Marathon attempt was nestled in between two big races, the London Marathon and my first ever attempt at a 100-mile event. The race, Thames Path 100, was a couple of weeks past Boston and the London Marathon was only the week before. The ultrarunner in me told me it was all good training and just to crack on. I would run London at a steady pace, allowing me to give Boston a go.

I saw a tweet from BBC newsreader Sophie Raworth. With a place in both London and Boston, she was asking the greater world which one she should do. I tweeted my response: 'Both! I am!'

I did not know her at all at the time, but I think now this was the answer she wanted to hear.

By sheer coincidence we happened to be on the same flight to Boston. We had a brief hello and chat and agreed to meet at the Race Expo to collect our bibs. Little did I know this encounter would lead to a running journey through many experiences, many races, miles of training runs and a close friendship that continues to this day.

This race became the catalyst for the meeting for a little group of runners who would egg each other on to another race, and then another. I wandered around the Expo with Sophie and Sam, London Marathon under our belt and still in our legs.

In there we became acquainted for the first time with a couple of other Brits, Ben Wickham and Tim Jones, also there for the marathon. We then happened upon a new area in the Expo: it was all blue and had 'Abbott World Marathon Majors' emblazoned all over it. I had never heard of such a thing. In the centre was a display featuring a huge medal. Sophie, rather like a magpie to shiny things, made straight for it.

This was the World Marathon Majors and we did not take very long to realise that it consisted of grouping together six of the biggest marathons in the world: New York, Chicago, Berlin, Tokyo, Boston and, yes, London. It hit us, both Sophie and me, that we were one day away from being a third completed. Next there was the 'Hall of Fame', a list of names of those who had finished all six races, and it was then that we realised that hardly any of the finishers were women. We both looked at each other. 'Well, that would be nice.'

Boston Marathon was tough. The course is so hard to pace correctly. The first 5 kilometres (3 miles) are downhill and I went through the distance two minutes over my 5K personal best – disastrous pacing – realising after checking my watch that I had just made the race even harder for myself. It was warm and hilly, and I found myself battling an internal monologue telling me to stop on the hills and walk.

This is Boston Marathon, Susie, Boston. You know how much you want to be here. RUN!

I managed to keep running, just, despite what the course threw at me. I wanted to do the race and myself justice.

I clung on as best I could, abandoning my Plan A of a personal best, and went for Plan B, which was to finish with another Boston qualifying time. Plan C (just finishing) nearly came into play up the infamous 'Heartbreak Hill' section, but I just managed to suck up the pain enough, and crossed the line with a full heart and terrible cramping legs.

This was one year after the horrifying bombing at the finish line. In 2013 two bombs were placed near the finish, detonating within seconds of each other, killing three people and injuring hundreds. At that point, there were nearly six thousand people still on the course, and the race was, of course, suspended. A year later, in 2014, people came back to Boston in their thousands to run and support the city. There was a determination to run and a heartfelt celebration for every single mile completed along the course that day.

A palpable air of emotion carried us runners through the distance. Everyone was proud to be part of the race. The motto *We Run As One* was emblazoned upon the race shirts; runners came together that day and set out to reclaim the finish line as their own. It was a huge privilege to be part of that field.

••••

With two of the majors ticked off, our little group of Brits gathered that evening over burgers and beers and vowed to keep going on the quest for the big Six Star medal. It was not going to be easy – and was also going to cost a fortune, which I absolutely did not have – but like Sophie, I wanted to see my name on that Hall of Fame list.

The easiest way to get entry to the World Marathon majors is to run a qualifying time. Which is not actually easy at all. With both London and the notoriously difficult-to-enter Boston done, our sights were set upon Berlin and New York.

New York had an entry time that I could just about scrape with a fast half-marathon, but Berlin's qualifying time was impossibly fast for me: I would have to run faster than 3 hours, 10 minutes. Impossible! I would have to cross my fingers for the ballot for that one and hope for the best.

Incredibly, I managed to tick both of them off quite quickly.

New York Marathon is the biggest race in the world. Over a million people line the streets as more than 50,000 runners take on the course that weaves you on a journey through all of New York's five boroughs. You have to be at the start line in Staten Island hours before the race kicks off, milling around in the November cold as the streets you are about to run through close to prepare. It's worth the wait! What a start!

As is customary in US races, the National Anthem signalled the final few minutes before the starting klaxon. Americans know how to express themselves – with whoops and air punches – and the atmosphere was buzzing with palpable anticipation as 'The Star-Spangled Banner' blared out over the crowd.

There was not a single cloud in the sky and the sun warmed my face against the chill. A helicopter was hovering overhead, a klaxon sounded and then we were off! Thousands of us headed out in formation, leaving Staten Island over the Verrazzano-Narrows Bridge. At this point, the course immediately sloped up. The sound of cheering, mixed with the buzzing of the helicopters and thousands of feet pounding the concrete, filled my ears. As I made my way to the crest of the bridge, New York in all its skyscraper glory rose into view ahead. Windows were twinkling in the early morning sun, the city stretched out as far as I could see, and I was about to run right through the heart of it.

The course was deceptively undulating, and the slopes of the bridges and shallow road gradients slowly took their toll on my quads. The gathered crowds got thicker, noisier and more boisterous with each borough until finally, when I turned off Madison Avenue Bridge, I was slapped by a wall of noise. Solid cheering, cowbells, music and clapping from a crowd of thousands made up the raucous cacophony that I could actually feel reverberating through me as I ran. The crowds and uphills continued all the way up Fifth Avenue until finally I turned into Central Park for the last couple of miles. With thousands of people yelling encouragement, music blasting and my fellow runners all suddenly running closer as the course narrowed, the whole experience felt so very amplified as I crossed a spine-tingling finish line. They say everything is bigger in America – and the New York Marathon really is an exceptional race.

Berlin is, by contrast, a different affair. The streets and views are a little less iconic, a little more pedestrian, but what it lacks in sights it makes up for in speed. It is a very fast course, a real runners' course. Efficient and straightforward, this was the scene for my marathon personal best. It was 2015, and I was in pretty good shape at the time and not expecting it, nor had I set out to run my fastest time. I was unlucky in the ballot, but fortunate enough to be invited by Adidas to take part. There had not been a huge amount of time to get marathon fit, yet by this stage in my running journey I was so deep into ultramarathons that the prospect of a marathon was neither intimidating nor difficult in terms of endurance running. I decided just to rock up to the start line, give it a go and see what happened. (How times had changed!)

The course was flat, the streets were wide, and as the crowds bunched together in the first few big long roads, it felt too crowded in parts, but the collective swell swept us along for the first few miles. Shaun joined me, having secured a place in the ballot, and he paced me like a metronome. I had gone in wanting sub 3:30 and as we moved along the course we hit every distance marker. The experience and endurance in my legs, coupled with the feeling of not being daunted by the distance, meant I felt very relaxed. The miles came and went without any drama and I felt good. By Mile 22, I knew I would be on for my fastest time. This only served to fuel me further. Encouraged by how good I was still feeling, I knuckled down to really focus on those last 4 miles. I ran my heart out, refusing to let my legs get slower, getting swept along, empowered by the knowledge I was running 26.2 miles faster than ever before for me. Then it was there in front of me, the majestic Brandenburg Gate. It signalled the last sprint for the finish line; driving my elbows back and pushing hard, I crossed it, breathing heavily but elated. This was and remains my fastest ever marathon. That night we went out celebrating and I accidentally got the most drunk I had been in years. Drinks appeared that I had not ordered and the night ended on a 'last nightcap' that went on for hours.

The next day I felt awful from the soles of my feet all the way up to the very top of my head. There was not a single part of me that did not feel the previous day's extravagance of miles and alcohol.

I returned to Berlin to run with Sophie the following year, both of us getting in via the ballot and wanting to run together.

At about seven in the evening the night before race day, I laid out all my kit on the floor to take a 'flat lay' picture to post on Instagram to show how race ready I was: race top, shorts, socks, race bib and trainers. It was only then that I realised I had bought two left feet trainers.

Not surprisingly, Berlin that year was a slightly different experience. I had to hurriedly borrow a pair of trainers, which were a whole size too small. Running along with Sophie was fun, but the second I crossed the finish line I could not bear the pain any longer, removed the too-small trainers and went back to the hotel in just my socks. I lost a few toenails that day.

••••

Having visited the Cat Café (stick-on whiskers and cat ears supplied upon entry) and the calm but impressive Imperial Palace, and eaten some of the freshest sushi on the planet, there was only one thing left to do in Tokyo. Run the marathon.

It was 2017, and I was there with Sophie and most of the Boston Marathon crowd: Tim, Sam, Ben and Emily Foy. Due to the time difference, we had made more of a holiday on this one, arriving a few days earlier to take in the bright lights of the culturally fascinating capital city, and were going to finish our mini-holiday in style by running 26.2 miles through it. Japan is probably my favourite travel destination, a mesmerising country where old traditions mingle seamlessly with the bright lights of pop culture. The city brims with people busying themselves in their work; they are a very industrious nation, yet they know how to make the most of their spare time. It would be typical to be in a Zen Japanese garden and then turn a corner and be almost overwhelmed with neon lights, kitsch anime and noisy pachinko gaming machines. And then there is running.

Running is like a religion in Japan. Runners are everywhere in the morning streets. Obediently stopping at pedestrian crossings, weaving their way through the web of roads into the calm sanctity of the temples and parks, finding time to run before work, before the streets fill up with commuters, workers, tourists.

We had gained 'sub-elite' entry by running what is known in other countries as 'Good For Age'. Tokyo would be our penultimate marathon on the quest for the World Marathon Majors, and it proved to be like no other with its politely joyful atmosphere, measured celebration and mutual respect – for each other and for the streets of Tokyo. As we made our way through the gleeful crowds clapping in an enthusiastic but contained way, not a single gel wrapper or water cup was dropped, nor was there even a single slight shove at drink stations.

Intriguingly, tomatoes, a uniquely Japanese race snack, appeared at every fuelling station. I tried one at about 16 miles in. It was neither too sweet nor too savoury and was strangely refreshing, even if it offered virtually no calorific benefit. Sophie and I ran together, she wearing a Union Jack vest which enticed more polite clapping and cries of 'Great Britain!'

The whole trip from start to finish was simply lovely. Our group finished the marathon content and happy. We had experienced a country so very different from our own; we had enjoyed being tourists, taken in as many sights as we could, experienced so many new and unfamiliar things, yet finished it doing something so very familiar.

We were all looking forward to collecting our Six Star Medal a few months later. Unbeknown to me, that final race in Chicago would bring a huge change for me, shattering my view on the world, how I ran and my self-confidence.

••••

Chicago Marathon 2017. *This is it. The culmination of a four-year quest to get our name on that Hall of Fame.*

I had been feeling rather strange off and on for several weeks. It was hard to put my finger on it. Nothing too pronounced or challenging, though running had become more difficult. I felt sluggish and tired a lot of the time. I was breaking into a sweat without much effort and found I was out of breath easily. Too much running? Getting older? A nasty cough a few months back had taken a hefty dose of antibiotics to shift and now, annoyingly, it had returned for marathon week.

Wanting to maximise the journey, Shaun and I had tagged on Detroit Marathon the week after Chicago. Detroit looked like a fun race and you need to carry your passport with you because the course takes you to Canada and back. With my daughter Lily in tow, the Six Star crowd met in Chicago. We were by now at slightly different stages of getting the big medal, but Sophie, Tim and I were to complete the Majors together after this race. Fitting because we had all started together in 2014 in Boston.

When the day before the marathon came round, my cough was so bad that I had to hold on to something or crouch down, such was the ferocity of the effort. It hurt my ribs, my throat and my lungs to cough. When I could feel the next cough coming, I had to brace myself. In a lift in a shopping centre, I started coughing and almost immediately people started pressing buttons to get out on the nearest floor. I sounded deathly.

'I'll be fine, I'll just take it steady.'

Wondering if there was anything I could do to make my marathon easier, I visited a pharmacy and was given cough medicine, which made me feel somewhat floaty and mildly drunk – kind of fun if you're not running a marathon. Filling pre-race time on activities which involved sitting down, we went on a tourist bus tour around the historic gangster haunts. I was full of cough medicine, somewhat woozy and laughing like a drain in the front seat. My daughter was rolling her eyes at me, but Tim found it hilarious.

As fun as the medication was – and it stopped the cough for an hour or so at a time – it was probably not one to take on race day.

Chicago is a massive race, with 40,000 people taking part. We set off down the huge skyscraper-lined avenues of the city, and I felt OK running at a steady pace and taking cough sweets. However, as the miles passed, things became a little hazier. I am usually a cheery participant, shouting and clapping back at the crowds, but this time I felt myself becoming weaker. I focused hard on the ground in front of me, and my mind and concentration started to cloud. I was sweating a lot and became very quiet. The cough was a problem. It was very difficult to run and cough at the same time.

I can remember leaning over to Sophie and telling her, 'If I faint, do not let them take me off the course. I have to finish. I simply have to finish.'

I made her promise me. I could not imagine coming so close to the end of the Six Star finish only to not make it, and have to wait a whole year to try again (assuming I could get in again).

I focused hard on keeping in step with those around me. At some point I noticed I was being closely flanked by Sophie on one side and Shaun on the other. Sideways glances were exchanged as I went mute with the effort of just getting through this.

The miles seemed to go on for an age, the distance on my watch creeping up by minute amounts every time I checked.

If you keep moving forward, you will eventually get to the finish line. This much I knew.

In the final half mile, the effort was really taking its toll and Sophie had hold of my hand. When we crossed the finish line, we both raised up our arms and were immediately funnelled to the Six Star Finish Area, where the giant medal was placed around our necks. From nowhere a camera crew showed up. The whole thing happened in a blur, but I was smiling and nodding, and looking at Sophie when they asked questions. All of a sudden, I started to see stars. Trying to blink them away, a blackness shrouded me, my head bowed and I knew I was going to faint.

A wave of Britishness took over me and I muttered a mild warning mixed with an apology, and promptly passed out.

I was still lying there on the ground just past the finish when I came round again to a circle of concerned faces. Embarrassed and not wanting a fuss, I apologised once again and then totally ruined Tim's own Six Star moment of glory. He crossed the line to find everyone looking at me in a heap on the floor.

Sophie gently ushered me to the medical tent to be checked over. Shaun waited outside while Sophie and I both sat in chairs, waiting to be attended to. With a bit of a fuss a few people came into the tent and a mildly hysterical lady was brought in and was promptly put on a drip.

I looked at Sophie and said: 'I'm not that bad' and got up to leave.

I was a bit sheepish about the whole episode. Sophie, bless her, helped me back to the hotel, insisted I have a hot bath and cup of sweet tea, and made me promise to call the doctor.

I have no idea how I got through the Detroit Marathon the following weekend feeling equally dreadful. It was a slow plod of an affair. I was sweating profusely and still with a hacking cough, but at least it gave me the opportunity to enjoy the marathon itself. It was a race full of heart and personality despite being considerably less fancy than Chicago.

••••

I called the doctor back in the UK, who heard me cough down the phone and booked me in for a chest X-ray the day I came back.

Two days later I got a call to come in for an ultrasound.

Two days after that I got a call saying I had sizeable growth in my neck.

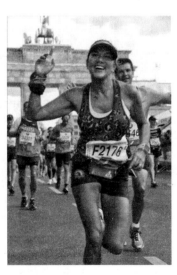

Closing in on a marathon PB in Berlin.

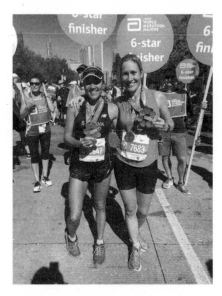

Berlin, Boston, London, New York, Tokyo and now Chicago.
With my dear friend Sophie as we became six-star
finishers – and just minutes before I fainted.

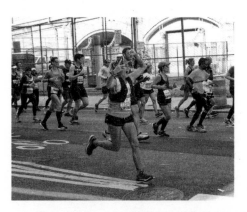

The biggest race in the world: running the New York Marathon in 2019.

10

THE HOSPITAL

Farnham hospital, November 2017

*'Surely there is nothing wrong with me? . . . I can
run 100 miles, for crying out loud.'*

I concentrate on staring at the ceiling.

The room is dimmed and the curtains closed so the sonographer
can see the screen on the ultrasound machine more clearly.

'Just tilt your chin up, look left.'

I focus hard on the corner of a ceiling tile in the grey light.

The cold gel is running round to the back of my neck and
I try to lie as still as possible.

He presses the probe quite hard into my neck and I can feel
my throat compressing with the pressure. He keeps on clicking
at his keyboard, eyes focused on his screen.

Turning my chin to the right as instructed, I try to catch
sight of the screen and make sense of it. How do they learn to
read these screens? How long does it take to make sense of the
information so they can just look at it and know what it is? It's
a series of black, white and grey random shapes, which mean
nothing to me. I watch out the side of my eye as he moves the
probe. He seems to be marking the screen with a series of lines,
perhaps measuring, clicking as he goes.

Other than giving me instructions on where to point my
chin, he says nothing at all.

*It's late Friday afternoon. Perhaps he's thinking about his weekend
already, what he has lined up for dinner.*

He keeps snapping away and pressing into my neck. It is not particularly comfortable and I suppress the urge to swallow in case it interferes with what he is doing.

Eventually, he stops prodding my neck and hands over some tissue. I wipe my neck, front and back, and sit up.

'Your doctor will be in touch.'

I generally try not to bother busy NHS people, and do not really know what's for the best in these situations, but I feel I have to ask. 'Everything OK?'

'I only do the ultrasound imaging and will share these with your doctor, who will be in touch soon, I am sure.'

Not unkind, but not really telling me anything.

I get up and get in my car and drive home, trying my best not to think about it.

••••

I had a lump around 7 cm long attached to my thyroid.

'These can happen and most commonly these are benign, nothing too much to worry about. Do you have any symptoms?' My GP was steady and calming.

I paused. It was really very hard to pinpoint anything in particular, but now I thought about it, there were several things that had been creeping up on me in the last few months. Could these all be connected? Were they symptoms?

I had been feeling sluggish a lot of the time. *Maybe it is the running*, I told myself.

I was hungry a lot of the time. *Probably the running.*

My weight had fluctuated and I was heavier. *You are just getting old, Susie.*

I was out of breath a lot more when I ran. *Not fit enough, train harder, Susie.*

I had a reason for all the small, little things that just did not make me feel like myself. However, now that I was really thinking about it, I was having to hang my tongue out like a puppy; it seemed to create more space to get the air in. *That's not normal. How long have I been doing that for?*

'Did you not notice it when you looked in the mirror?'

Now I could not unsee it. Clearly visible, pushing through the skin in my neck, the lump did look quite large. I examined myself in the mirror that night, turning my chin one way and the other, holding my chin up while looking down my nose in the mirror to see if I could spot any difference. No wonder I was having trouble breathing, said the doctor.

I got sent to a different hospital, where a clearly busy Ear, Nose and Throat doctor gave my notes a cursory look over, prodded my neck with his fingers, told me to take some Gaviscon and if it got bigger to let them know. The whole appointment was over in four minutes.

••••

Something inside told me that this did not feel right at all. *Besides, how am I supposed to be able to keep running like this?*

Now I was aware of it, it was really bothering me. A bit like when you have a tiny pain on your hand, then look and see a paper cut, at which point it becomes more sore.

Then there was the fact that I had lots of races over the next few months, flights had been booked and everything. I wanted a second opinion and returned to my doctor.

My GP could not fail to hide how livid she was that nothing further had been done, considering the size of the lump.

••••

I stared at the ceiling, this time in a different room in London. The doctor held what looked like a slim knitting needle in one hand and told me to relax. I tried to relax my chest and shoulders, but clenched my hands into fists as he leaned over me and placed the point of the needle right in the middle of my throat. I could feel the nails of my hands pressing into my palms as he pierced the skin with the needle.

'We will be looking for a certain shape of the cell,' he told me. As he was talking, I was trying to listen to the words and absorb them, but in the end I could not remember if having a comet-shaped cell in the biopsy was a good or a bad thing. As he was chatting away, trying to keep things light, I lay there and started to realise what was actually happening. Suddenly my mind started racing in all directions; up until now I had been floating through this experience in a mild state of denial. Yet now, with a needle inches into my neck, listening to the word 'biopsy', I could not quite grasp a single thought long enough to carry it through before another one shot into my mind.

Surely there is nothing wrong with me?
I am only 42 years of age, I can run 100 miles, for crying out loud.
This is absurd.
Lily . . .

All of the doctors, every single one of them, had told me lumps were very common in the thyroid.

'Generally fine.'

'Common thing to happen.'

'Not likely cancer.'

Apparently, lumps are more common in women. Asians also tend to get them. As do people in their forties. I was slap bang in the middle of the Venn diagram.

••••

A different doctor this time. No ceiling to stare at because he was sitting opposite me behind a very tidy desk.

He had a serious face with kind eyes and an air of professionalism and efficiency that made me trust him straight away.

Sophie was with me. She had raced here directly from the newsroom. 'I can help you take the information in.' She once again held my hand.

The results were inconclusive – very likely to be benign, but really the only way to know was to have the lump removed.

He did say that in his opinion it was very large and that it would be for the best to have it taken out given that it was starting to obstruct my airway.

'This is good, Suse! It is progress!'

On the way out Sophie bought me a sandwich from the hospital shop. She was of course right. She always is. *This is a good thing. Get it removed and I can breathe and run again!*

Neither of us mentioned the fact that we were supposed to be heading out to the Marathon des Sables in two months' time, a huge race for Sophie and one she had dreamed of, trained extremely hard for and had kept secret from everyone. We were planning on going together and enjoying it together by running all the way together.

••••

The anticipation of knowing you are about to start a long, difficult race, and knowing you are about to have an operation are very similar feelings. You know what is about to happen, you have accepted it, accepted that you are likely to get hurt but will come out on the other side, recover and then feel good.

My surgeon, a very dashing, handsome doctor called Mr Ofo, reassured me that this was his speciality. He was an expert in removing thyroid lumps. The risks of surgery affecting your windpipe and breathing ability include damage to your vocal cords, which can affect your voice because everything in that part of your neck sits very close to each other.

'Try not to worry, you will be fine.'

His soothing deep voice with an air of clear control and authority softened the edges of my fear.

••••

The smiling eyes above the hospital mask spoke to me. 'I'm going to count down from 10, and you will drop off.'

I looked up at the ceiling, once again focusing on the corner of a tile. Within seconds, I was out.

When I came round, the first thing I was aware of was a tube coming out of the middle of my neck. My head seemingly was made of lead and I could not seem to move it, so my eyes followed where the tube went – down the side of the hospital bed, out of view. I could not speak. I had a very sore throat, and even the thought of speaking seemed like an effort. Just the notion of saying a word caused the muscles in my voice box to flex slightly – which hurt.

The grogginess wore off slowly. I was tired and drifted in and out of sleep for a day. My voice slowly started to return in whispers as nurses came and went looking after me.

••••

My phone rang. 'Do you want anything?'

'Ice cream,' I whispered.

Sophie turned up later that day holding a freezer bag with litres and litres of ice cream in all sorts of flavours. I was not at all hungry but ate small bits of the ice cream, one slow teaspoon at a time, which soothed and cooled my neck from the inside.

After two days it was time to leave. Mr Ofo came in to see me and he was very happy with my progress.

'I can see why it was giving you trouble. Sometimes these lumps can be quite soft, but this was one quite hard to touch. Want to see a picture?'

Curiosity made me look.

The photo showed the offending article laid out on a green fabric on a surgical tray. It was next to a small measuring tape and had grown more since my last scan.

As I looked at it, I could feel the strange slight pang within the empty space now left in my neck.

'We will send it off to Histology and I will be in touch with the results. We just need to remove the tube from your neck and you can head home to rest up more.'

With another dazzling smile and encouraging nod, he left me with a nurse.

The tube had not been too troubling unless I accidentally tugged on it or knocked it with an elbow. Having it removed was not something I particularly wanted, yet it had to be removed for me to go home. Telling me to breathe in and exhale slowly, the nurse pulled it out with three sharp movements. It was much, much longer than I expected, which shocked me a little. With each tug I felt the sensation of it being pulled from somewhere deep within my neck, between the skin and the windpipe. It was full of a bloody, yellow liquid. This was not too painful, but the whole thing made me tense, which hurt. It was such an unsettling and alien feeling, I nearly vomited, which in turn made me scrunch my eyes and fists up in pain.

••••

I slept a lot in the next couple of days and tried to go out for a very short walk with my dogs. The slit in my throat was stitched up nicely, but it felt so terribly bruised and the muscles all around my neck ached deeply. It was hard to swallow and I could feel the wound on the inside.

Not until you are unable to move something do you realise how much you use it. Even the slightest, most subtle turn of the head hurt, so I would turn my body slowly by the shoulders or at the waist or try to look at things out of the side of my eyes.

My neck was still sore and swollen, and I did not feel well within myself, weak and thick in my movements. The prescribed painkillers were just about doing enough to target the wound, but everything else felt terrible. Not just my neck but my whole body. As the days passed my neck did not seem to be any less sore or any less inflamed. If anything, it seemed to be getting bigger and I was starting to feel worse again.

Is this normal? It was surgery, after all; of course there would be swelling and soreness.

After five days of no improvement, still feeling awful and with terrible neck pain, things continued to get worse and not better. I was having trouble holding my own head up and at times resorted to using my hands to rest it or prop it up, giving my neck muscles a rest. *This is horrendous. Perhaps I could use some stronger medication?*

I thought about phoning the hospital and then, suddenly, within the space of a couple of hours my neck had swollen dramatically under the bandages.

Shaun drove me back to the hospital where Mr Ofo worked. He was on holiday with his family, but the nurses looked at me and very quickly decided to call him up on his holiday.

After some hushed conversations, Mr Ofo called me directly on my mobile phone. 'You need to go to A&E immediately.' He directed me to a nearby hospital where his colleague would be waiting.

After a drive in which I started to feel increasingly unwell and had to hold my head in my hands, we arrived to a full A&E department and a queue at the front desk to check in. I had to sit down, feeling terrible and really needing to rest my head on something.

Thankfully, we were not there for very long. A doctor came through the reception calling my name and ushered me swiftly in to an adjacent room.

He was on the phone to Mr Ofo simultaneously.

I lay down on the bed as directed and he peeled back my dressings.

There was a cricket-ball sized lump on my neck and the scar was weeping heavily.

He silently stared hard at it for a long few seconds.

I started to feel frightened.

Things happened rather quickly after that. The doctor performed an emergency draining on my neck, going straight in and making a small incision with a scalpel as I lay there gripping the sides of the hospital bed. I had my eyes closed and can remember feeling lots of foul-smelling fluid coming out, dripping down on my neck and shoulders, the doctor mopping it up with tissues. Shaun was in the room, looking at me with serious concern, and he wordlessly grabbed hold of my hand.

The wound seemed almost immediately to fill back up again.

The doctor walked into a corner and had another conversation on the phone.

I was readmitted to the hospital, but after a few hours things had still not improved. Shaun stayed until they told him he had to leave, so he slept in the car in the car park, hoping to be let back in as soon as the ward opened.

I was monitored overnight and in the morning a doctor came around to speak to me. All the while she was talking to me her eyes wandered down to my neck and back to my face to talk to me.

'I don't want another operation,' I feebly requested.

Her eyes settled back on my neck. She was kind, but firm.

Very shortly after this I was whisked into theatre for an emergency operation and once again my neck was cut open.

••••

When I came around, I can vividly remember feeling so much better, brighter. Yes, my neck was sore, but my general feeling of being unwell, of fighting some deep-set illness, had gone. I noticed I felt hungry for the first time in a week.

A few hours later, without asking for permission, I gingerly ventured in search of food. I held on to my hospital gown to stop it unravelling and took the lift down to an M&S near the hospital entrance. Not wanting to get told off for disappearing, I stood in a corridor near my ward eating a cheese sandwich slowly when Mr Ofo, fresh off a plane, wandered past. He had come to see me.

'I feel much better!'

'I can see!'

He was glad; mine had been an extremely rare complication and I was to take it easy after this. Histology results would be back in two weeks.

••••

There was a work gig scheduled for later in the week. Being self-employed by this point, it was a great opportunity that I did not want to miss. I had agreed to it months ago, and as the date approached I assumed I would be comfortably on the road to recovery and, at the very least, able to walk fine. It was a photo shoot for a big sports brand, which involved them coming to my home and filming me, followed by a trip out to a countryside venue and some running shots. These shoots generally tend to involve an awful of standing around, a bit of posing and short bursts of running. Totally manageable, I'd assumed, plus the pay was good and I needed the money.

Since the second operation, I was feeling so much better, apart from a really achy and still sore neck, which meant that head movement was still not possible. But I was sleeping and moving around better. OK, I wasn't sure if I could run, and reasonably certain that if I asked Mr Ofo for his permission he would say no. So I simply didn't ask.

The film crew rolled up and with supreme efficiency we captured a lot of standing and smiling and lifestyle photos and videos. Ideally I wanted to keep my recovery a secret, worried that they would otherwise suddenly pack up and leave, or judge me as not fit enough for the job.

It dawned on me that there was no way we would get through this without everyone knowing. I had planned on removing the dressing on my neck just before anyone showed up and not drawing any attention to my neck. Of course, when I did this, there was a very fresh wound – with stitches and still weeping and clearly not very photogenic at all. I do not know what I was thinking.

I told the director straight away who was nothing but kind and told me not to worry at all.

I was handed a variety of clothes, including a jacket to wear for one particular photo. It had a high neck, so we all thought that would be the best thing to start off with. Zipping it all the way up to my neck, I bled on to it within seconds. I was mortified, but they had another.

When it came to running, I had barely walked since the operation, so was very worried about how it would feel. *Will I have any energy? Will the wound open up again? Is this going to hurt? Is everyone on this set talking about me and my weeping neck?*

The running section was filmed at Box Hill, infamous among cyclists and trail runners alike because of its steep climbs, and the director selected a long uphill section for me to run up and down.

I must be hiding it well, I thought. Up and down the road I ran, smiling, trying to look athletic and focused. They snapped and filmed away as I did my best to hold it together. As time wore on I became very tired, not run tired but tired from deep within.

'Just one more shot and we are done!'

Thank god for that. I smiled and ran some more and they got all the content they needed.

'That's a wrap! Thank you, Susie.'

••••

Three months later the campaign went live, and I was in shops and advertisements all over Europe and the US. I was sent an image by another runner of a huge backlit advertising hoarding at the start of the Manchester Marathon. The tag read:

'SUSIE CHAN, Endurance Runner and Supermum.'

Looking at it, you could not tell that I just had an operation, that I was clinging on to my smile, trying to look good. *Fake it till you make it.*

••••

The results came back: a papillary thyroid carcinoma. The most common thyroid cancer and the most easily treatable. I see other people going through their cancer journeys and know that mine was straightforward. There were discussions about possible follow-up treatments, but it was decided overall that monitoring was the best approach. I had only a small part of my thyroid left, but it seemed to be picking up the slack. The risk was back to normal. I was very lucky, aware that others are less so, and that many endure long and gruelling treatment journeys. I decided not to dwell on things, not wanting to really speak about too much or make too much of it. I wanted to just crack on as quickly as possible with my life.

I wonder now if there was a part of me that needed to prove to myself I was well again, that my body was capable of doing the same thing as before. Up until this point it had always been able to do what I had demanded of it: run faster, run further, be tougher.

I threw myself into all the races planned. First up, just two weeks after the second operation, was the Big Half in London: 13.1 miles around the streets finishing at the *Cutty Sark*. I went along to the start and decided I would take it very easy and get moving again. If I needed to stop, I told myself, I would.

In a similar cadence to my very first half-marathon, I set out unsure of how far I would get, how long would it be before I became tired. With each passing mile the crowd grew and got thicker, as did the cheering, the smiles and the energy. I could feel it nourishing me. It was a pure, palpable joy. I felt the running, the thrill of being part of the community, revive and invigorate me. I sailed across the finish line with the hugest smile on my face. Sophie, who had also run the event, was waiting for me at the *Cutty Sark,* eyes on the finish line, looking for me. There is something about being part of an enormous event that is so simple. We turn up, we run together, we celebrate.

••••

I had been in hospital in February and racing again by March, and it was not even a consideration for me not to keep training for my next two events. In May I would take on an energy-sapping 100-mile race, running the entire distance of the Florida Keys. More pressingly in April I would be heading out once again to the Marathon des Sables – this time with my friend, the person who had supported me from that very first fainting episode in Chicago, to holding my hand in appointments, to calling me, checking in, keeping my spirits up and bringing me ice cream. Sophie was off to do the Marathon des Sables; she had been training like a demon and there was no way in the world I was going to not be there to see her fulfil her race dream. Neither of us needed to say it: she knew it, I knew it, we were off.

Once again, the desert awaits.

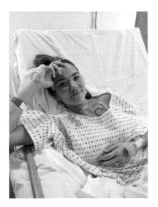

Recovering in hospital.

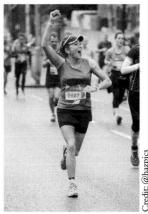

Just two weeks after my second operation, I was back racing the Big Half in London. The joy of running alongside thousands of others was thrilling and nourishing.

11

'HAVE A WORD WITH YOURSELF'

Marathon des Sables, 2017 and 2018

'You have ups and downs, keep going!'

What is the point?

No seriously? Why am I doing this? It's shite. Maybe I should just stop. I'm gaining nothing from being here. Nothing.

I look at my feet. The gaiters are caked in sand, I can see holes in them already, I can feel my feet clammy and slightly swollen, toes pressing on the ends of the trainers.

Sitting down in the shade of a Land Rover, I contemplate my options. *Withdraw from the race. That would be nice. Just getting in a car back to Camp and not having to run another step in this stupid fucking desert. Or carry on.* There are only two options.

I look up. Runners are passing through the checkpoint, some pouring their rationed water over their faces, over their arms. Some laugh, chat. They're focused, tired but content. Happy to be here. *That was me once.*

They go past me, step around me and between the dirty white Land Rovers and head back out into the sand once more, a line of runners snaking out into the horizon for as long as I can see, into the hot dunes.

I do not want to be here. I came along by myself, fortunate enough to be invited back by the race organisers, mentioned as 'one to watch' after my last race, which saw me snapping at the fringes of the elites. Now, two years later, here I am, sitting down, feeling petulant despite the huge privilege of the opportunity, feeling broken emotionally, with not an ounce of enthusiasm.

I stare, unfocused, towards my feet. 'Have a word with yourself,' I mutter aloud.

I watch as others who have grafted, trained and saved their way to be here continue on in the race of their dreams, and it occurs to me what an utter asshole I am.

I get up and head back out into the dunes.

••••

My preparation for this race could not have been further from my first time. The calculated, methodical approach of 2015 has gone, the fitness has waned. After two successful races, I came in to this one so disorganised that I was buying race food at Pret a Manger in Gatwick Airport. *Nuts? They could work. Crisps? Perfect for breakfast Day 1.*

I went into my race bags and dug out my miniature and trusted matchbox-sized stove, found my old venom pump, dusted off my rucksack. An invitation! How flattering! Me! *Give it a go. What's the worst that can happen?*

Being less fearful of failure meant I was setting myself up for it.

While I had all the right equipment to hand, and I could pull together race food and clothes from what I had in cupboards and wardrobes, what I had neglected, not even thought about, was my reason to run for days through the desert again.

Having a reason to run the race, whatever it is – from a 5K to an ultramarathon – will get you through the most challenging parts and to the finish line. You need a reason to be there, a why, and as I trudged slowly through the stage, feet dragging in the heavy sand, lips burnt crisp from the sun's rays, it became crystal clear to me that apart from being flattered to be invited, I had none.

I had come alone and knew a few of the runners. I was lucky enough to be in a tent together with really talented and easy-going people.

I went out on Day 1 like a rocket, full of attitude and confidence. *I know this race. I understand how it pans out. I know the lie of the land. I was on the periphery of the elites last time, no less!* My pack felt heavy with the burden of the week's food, tugging at my shoulders with each step, but still I ran the stage hard, *too* hard. By Day 2 my energy ground to a halt and so did my enthusiasm.

Back in Camp, others were all chatting about their day, and what had worked. I stayed silent and when asked, just said I was not in a great place.

Remembering Shaun struggling for days last time, I thought there might be something wrong with me, so trudged over to the medical tent for the first time ever in the race.

The doctors cast their gaze over me, and gave me nothing but a few nice but firm words and a camp bed to lie down on. Giving me anything would have meant a time penalty; they save drips, extra bottles of water and medication for those in need, not for those with bruised egos. I just lay there in the medical tent for 30 minutes, feeling miserable and sorry for myself, and secretly enjoying not lying down on a rocky floor in a sweaty sleeping bag.

I felt a little embarrassed. I had imploded so hard after going out too quickly, a classic runner's error. My tent had two elites in it, Nathan Montague and Damian Hall, both cruising along and having a great race. I woke up each morning to Damian's polite and mild-mannered chatter, and Nathan doing pistol squats to warm up – the only person who could get away with doing something like that and still be charming.

I had been full of confidence, relaxed and even vaguely dismissive about the difficulty of the race. Having run it twice and also been through the jungle, I thought it would be relatively easy.

Oh, how wrong I was. I was not as fit, as organised or as focused as the last time. I came to the desert expecting an easy ride and the desert had other ideas.

Out of the medical tent, I ambled back to my tent, where people said soothing things and of course did not judge me at all.

Tomorrow would be the long stage. Normally I would be looking forward to getting my teeth into it. The long stage means you are edging ever closer to the finish line. It's the one where ultrarunners can really push themselves and in the past I have enjoyed the challenge. Not this time. I could feel the dread settling into my stomach as I tried to sleep. I could not get over the feeling that I just did not want to be here anymore.

The stage started much like the others. Avoiding talking to anyone, I set out. Trudging through the stage, one slow rocky mile after the other, I thought about a conversation with Sophie, agreeing to take on the race with her the following year, in 2018. In fact, we were already booked in. With every step under the scorching hot sun, I thought about being back here in one year's time, with a friend, and not out trudging on my own, feeling sorry for myself and empty. Trouble was, I kept returning to that thought – in the knowledge that I would be back in 12 months – and it made the whole thing seem even more pointless. I thought about stopping again; over and over I played out the sequence of events if I stopped. What I would say to people.

The next time I hit a checkpoint, I went over and told someone I was not enjoying it at all. The Doc Trotter medic looked at me and patted me on the shoulder: 'You have ups and downs, keep going!'

They were well versed in saying positive things and doing everything possible to keep people in the race. I rejoined the line of runners and tried everything I could to try not to think about how slowly I was moving, and how far there was still to go, and how much I was hating every single step.

I was lost in the self-indulgence of my own misery when a voice cut through: 'Hey, Susie!'

I turned around and a tiny, friendly blonde woman smiled at me. 'Mind if I join you for a bit? It's really warm and think I am going to walk for a while.'

Catrin Tyler was about to turn my race around for me.

We started to chat and march in a steady rhythm. She was witty and easy-going and made me feel good about my somewhat dreadful pace up until now.

The hours and miles passed by, more quickly now, and I realised the simple distraction of company had made the whole day much more positive.

As the sun set once again in a dazzling fanfare of pinks, oranges and purples, the temperature cooled.

'I think I might push on if that's OK?'

The fact she had even asked was kind. 'Have a great run!'

I watched as her tiny frame, dwarfed by her huge rucksack, sped off strong ahead of me as I continued my trudge – and was very grateful. Grateful for the conversation, the friendship and the miles shared.

I continued into the night, fighting off the DNF demons as best I could. If I finished this stage, there would be only the marathon distance to go – *and I can grind out a marathon, I know I can, it's something that I've managed several times before. Just keep going, Susie, one foot in front of the other.*

With a bit more spring in my step and a bit more focus, I made it through those last isolated and lonely miles to the long stage finish line. It could not come quickly enough that day.

••••

A new day. The 'rest day' because I had managed to complete the long stage in one go. Although my spirit was deflated, my muscles and legs felt OK. This was a win of some description.

You are not allowed a phone in Camp and the only real form of communication comes via messages sent to you from home. These are delivered in the evening to each tent, and the messages are at least 24 hours old by then, having been printed out, sorted into piles that correspond with surnames and tent numbers, and delivered.

Those messages are a highlight. Maybe it's that you are in the middle of a desert and isolated from the world, maybe it's that you cannot just pick up a phone to chat, maybe it's the day-on-day tiredness, but those messages give you an emotional high. Every kind word is felt and amplified, meaning is found in simple sentences, encouragement taken to heart.

The rest day messages were delivered, and I read through heaps of them from friends and people I had never met. Lots of words of encouragement; people had noticed I had dropped right back and were now telling me that I was doing great! Keep going! Nothing you have not done before! As well as the encouraging words, there were jokes and stories from the news, riddles to solve.

As I read through them, it dawned on me that my sluggishness was, in fact, a serious case of sulking. There was nothing wrong with me other than wounded pride. I had gone out too quickly, misjudged my fitness and not been prepared. Since then I had wallowed in this seeming failure. Yet how lucky I was to be there, in this beautiful environment, surrounded by like-minded and inspiring people, many of whom had trained and cared as much as I had done for that very first race.

I felt humbled, and embarrassed all over again, this time for a different reason. The chance of doing well in any placing was gone, but I did have one more day out here in the Marathon des Sables, which was once the biggest dream I had. As I lay there, sweltering in the tent, my eyes went from the pile of messages to the landscape around me: the mountains, the dunes in the distance, the changing colours of the sky. *Tomorrow is the marathon stage, and I will give the Sahara the respect it deserves and run like this is the last run of my life.*

••••

The elites cheered us off as we ran under the white starting arch to the familiar sound of AC/DC blaring out 'Highway to Hell' and for the first time in several days I felt happy. Running really is simple: you run as best you can on the day and that is all you can do. There is only being the best you can be on the day. A lighter pack bounced around on my shoulders as I ticked off the miles for the final time – for this year at least. It was not easy, it was still a struggle, but with each mile that passed I could feel my confidence grow, and a warmth and appreciation for running return.

I could see the finish line from a long way away. As it grew larger with my approach, I thought about how this race was different, how I had not enjoyed it, and how important it is in these events to have good people around you. This race has always been for me about those around me, the company I keep. You can look at a beautiful sunset and appreciate it, but you can look at a beautiful sunset with someone and enjoy it more. The experience is amplified if you see it with someone else; experiences are so much better shared.

I thought about this, about how much this race meant to me, and how I had come into it with the wrong focus. The truth was that I was never going to place well: I simply had not trained well enough, committed myself. Running has never really been about getting a good ranking for me – nice as that is, it is not what drives me. As I have continued in my running journey, the best runs, the ones I thought about when I thought of my favourite runs, were not the ones where I was chasing down minute miles, trying to keep pace. The best runs were the ones with my friends, with great views, where what I remembered was not the finish time but the scenery, the conversations, the laughs and the people I met. Those runs were the ones I cherished, the ones I will take with me to old age.

I crossed the line of the 2017 Marathon des Sables once again with a huge smile on my face.

The desert had been harsh to me this time around, but it had taught me an invaluable lesson.

••••

Sophie had barely said a word since we had left. The caravan of coaches was winding its dusty path from Ouarzazate south to the now-familiar landscape of the western side of the Sahara. I was babbling away, chatting to everyone, excited to be here – a very different feeling from last year. Now I was with a small and tight group of friends and the excitement was the kind when you have something fun, interesting and impressive that you want to show off to your friends. I could not wait to get to Camp.

I was leaning forward chatting to those two seats in front, and then turning round talking to those in the seats to my right, in the seats behind. Sophie stayed fixed, staring out the window.

'I'm very out of my comfort zone,' she said after a while in a voice so quiet it was barely audible.

'Oh, you'll be fine! It's so much FUN!'

She said nothing again.

We had been training together – secretly because she didn't want anyone to know – for months. We had taken in marathons, 50 miles along the North Downs Way, and hundreds of miles along trails. Anytime I mentioned Marathon des Sables in the first few months, I was met with silence, and I started to wonder if she wanted to do it at all, though she doggedly got all the training done.

Then I became unwell with cancer in the months leading up to the race. I had just had an operation when Sophie ran a multistage ultra, one we were supposed to run together: a great training race along the Pilgrims' Way through the Surrey Hills. After completing 66 miles of mud and covering thousands of feet of elevation, she came directly from the finish line, still muddy and unchanged, to my house to see me and check how I was doing.

So there really was not any question in my mind that I would not make the start line that year. Every year at the Marathon des Sables there are people there who defy medical issues and showcase ability over disability. Kevin Webber, diagnosed with prostate cancer and initially given only months to live, returns to the desert year after year, defying medical predictions. I have toed the start line with blind runners, wondering how they ascend and descend the sharp rocks of technical climbs which make the sighted stumble. I have seen athletes scaling Saharan sand dunes with one leg, no legs, no arms. My one recent and very treatable cancer episode really was nothing spectacular in the Marathon des Sables. We are all the same on that start line. All there to have our own race with the desert and not each other.

Only when we were a couple of weeks out, and sitting together making final decisions on our kit, did I confirm to myself that it was simply too late to back out now.

We went through the kit item by item. 'What about this?' Sophie asked, holding up something – a thin top, flip-flops, a battery pack.

'Do you really need it? Is it completely necessary?'

'I think so.'

'"Think"? It's a no.'

Some items made the cut, many did not. Slowly we had got our pack weight down, finalising what to bring, and I was getting excited. A week in the desert, doing the thing I love, running, in a place I love with my friends! Exciting! Sophie was more nervous than excited, and it occurred to me my boundless enthusiasm for this race might be slightly annoying, but I could not help it.

••••

On the coach the roadbook was handed out just as it had been three times before for me. As well as Sophie, I was there with two friends both called Tim, a new friend called Oli, and Shaun, who had returned to try to put some heat-running demons to bed, and find some sort of redemption.

We opened up the roadbook and fortunately it threw up no real surprises. Textbook racing for days; three days in a row shorter than marathon distance, one of the three was more technical; then the ultramarathon stage; and as ever finishing on a marathon.

After last year's harsh and humbling lesson, this year was all about sharing the experience. Sophie and I vowed to stick together.

Upon arrival in Camp, everyone relaxed into Camp life. Jokes were cracked, snacks were consumed, and the order in which we lay in the tent decided, everyone having their own reasons for their choice. The middle meant you had the use of the central pole, the edges meant a bit more privacy. No spots could guarantee things not being blown away by sudden gusts of desert wind.

Sophie and I wandered around a couple of tents meeting fellow runners, and then found the camel handlers to take photos with them. People were orientating themselves around Camp; there was a quiet buzz and a sense of expectation. When it was time for us to be processed, we headed into the huge admin tent, surrendered our luggage and emerged out the other side with nothing but our full rucksacks and our good spirits.

On the first morning of the first day, after waiting for a considerable amount of faffing about in the tent which would turn out to be the morning norm, we assembled on the start line to watch Patrick dad dancing, sing 'Happy Birthday' to several people and be blasted with AC/DC. The sun shone hard in a spotlessly blue sky. With heavy packs, bright white clean gaiters Velcroed to our trainers, and full bottles of water secured to our fronts, we headed out under the start arch for the first time.

••••

Day 1 was a bit of everything and a manageable 18 miles. It turned out to be gloriously uneventful in that no one overheated, everyone took it steady and we all finished feeling pretty good. We had stayed together – Sophie, myself, Shaun and one of the Tims (Tim D), forming a little quartet of ultrarunners, falling in step with each other effortlessly. We balanced each other out, one of us bolshy and bold, one quiet and consistent, one sensible and determined, and me, likely annoyingly peppy, but still fitting in. We were happy to chat about everything, yet equally comfortable with long silences, moving through the miles, up and down dunes, stepping in time with each other.

After finishing the stage on that first evening, we sat together in a line facing the sunset and preparing our evening meal: the usual array of rehydrated fodder, noodles and rice. People assessed their feet, repacked their bags, sorted their nutrition out for the next stage – tent mates establishing their night-time routines which helped us settle for the night.

•••

The next two stages were longer, sandier and more technical. They included our first ascent of my personal nemesis, the Jebel El Otfal. I had warned everyone about my fear of this climb, my uselessness with heights. Having conquered it before, I was not as fearful as previous years, and my thoughts turned to my friend Tim J, whose phobia of heights was much more chronic. By then, he and I had covered several of the World Marathon Majors together; we both used to joke about how much we hated heights, sending each other short videos from the internet of people skydiving in precarious situations, diving off huge cliffs into the sea, or teetering on the edge of mountains to get the Instagram shot.

'Fools!'

'Look at this absolute wrong 'un.'

'I just could not!'

Only in Chicago for the marathon the previous year did I realise just how severe his fear was. We had gone to the Willis Tower, famous for its Skydeck, a glass box that hangs on the side of the skyscraper offering tourists far-reaching views of the city. Tim had said he wanted to come along, but was not sure he would go up the skyscraper due to his fear of heights. We cajoled him into coming into the lift, telling him he could just stay on the normal floor area of the building, and not step into the Skydeck. I wasn't sure I would go near it either.

As the elevator doors slid open, Tim went white as a sheet and started to panic. Windows spanned all of the walls around us and we were over 1300 feet up in the air, on the 103rd floor with panoramic city views in every direction. He was rooted to the spot, people pushing past him, asking him to get out of the way.

I grabbed his arm and we were out on to the main floor. He was wide-eyed and fearful, but something inside him made him want to edge, one small shuffle at a time, to the windows, to the Skydeck.

'I think I want to go in it,' he declared.

Christ, that means I'll have to also.

He took a while, but he made it all the way gingerly to the edge of the glass box. By this point people all around were noticing what a huge effort this was, and in that American way, were all encouraging him.

'You got this, buddy!'

'You can do it!'

He refused to look down and with the tiniest, smallest of steps put his toes on the edge of the glass.

'One more step, buddy!'

'Awesome! You are crushing it!'

He looked at me and said, 'Get the camera ready.'

I held up my phone as he took the one step into the Skybox, hundreds of feet up, petrified and smiling.

Everyone cheered and I took the photo.

He could not get out of the building quick enough, but was buzzing when we finally made it back down to the sidewalk.

••••

On the morning of the Jebel climb day, I watched as Tim J walked away from the tent by himself and stopped several metres away from Camp, facing outwards to the mountains that lay ahead. Mountains we were about to go over.

I left him for a few minutes, then after a while walked out to join him. He had his sunglasses on, but I could see a tear trickle down his cheek.

'Big day today.'

'You are going to be brilliant. You can do it, Tim.'

'I want to finish this race.'

'You will.'

I thought about Tim J as we scaled up the Jebel, our group of four. I found courage thinking about him, knowing he would have to find the strength within himself to get up and, more terrifyingly, over the top. I thought about how he must have been feeling for the entire day and the days before, right until the moment the climb was there ahead of him.

This was also going to be the first time Sophie experienced the climb, having heard only my slightly hysterical reviews of how steep and high it is.

Sophie, a confident and accomplished skier, had no concerns or issues at all scaling and descending the mountain. Technical terrain did not seem to bother her. She was much stronger than me in this regard, helping me along and up shallower mountains. We climbed up and threw ourselves over the top. Arms in the air, all smiles on the rapid descent. After we had made the sandy run down and the course flattened out, she said, 'God help Tim on that.'

We both hoped he would make it.

Back in Camp we waited for his return. Each time we saw someone who looked like it could be Tim J, we strained our eyes, trying to find familiarity in the walk, the clothes.

Time passed and he did not return. We were starting to try to calculate a reasonable window for a finish time for him, when we heard, 'WASSUP, BITCHES! Here he is! He made it!'

Oli Lurot announced Tim J's return.

We gave him the hero's welcome he deserved. He was exhausted yet euphoric. Oli and Tim had stayed together as Tim made slow but persistent progress up to the top of the Jebel. Once he had reached the peak, the view and sharp descent made his legs feel like jelly, so he came shuffling down the other side on his bum, arms either side stabilising him, staying like this the whole way, picking his route down while staying as low as possible.

'Honestly, I have so much sand in my shorts I could build a sandcastle,' he said with a huge grin of accomplishment on his face. We were all delighted for him.

For most people climbing up and running over that mountain was just another exciting part of the race. A mountain climb can be easy for one person and be so much more to someone else. Achievements are personal; you can never really tell what courage it has taken for someone to get through a challenge. There are little personal battles being overcome, fought against and completed all around us. Little fears, little wins, everywhere, every day. Everyone has their own reasons to come to the desert and as far as Tim J was concerned, he had already won.

••••

'Wassup, bitches' became our daily greeting to each other. Oli Lurot was hilarious company. Loud, gregarious and self-deprecating, he would squat outside the tent smoking the occasional cigarette, making us all roar with laughter every morning – setting us up for the day with a smile on his face.

The long stage was 53 miles this year. Significant mileage with big climbs in the first half and a sea of sand dunes in the second.

The hunger had set in by Day 4. We were weary in our bones from the rough sleeping, our kit was thick with salt and dirt. Nothing was clean – our kit, our sleeping bags, our hair, our skin.

A sandstorm had whipped through Camp overnight. We had tried our best to hold up the poles to keep our shelter overhead, until the wind won the battle and the rough black fabric of the tent enveloped us in a dusty darkness, filling our nostrils and sleeping bags with sandy dust. We collectively resigned ourselves to this gritty, thick shroud in an unspoken agreement, all just lying passively underneath it while the wind whistled loudly around us, whipping and snapping at the corners of the fabric. Around Camp, over the whistling wind, we could hear poles falling, people crying out, yelling instructions to each other in French and English to try to maintain some sort of cover from the elements. We remained in a tight pile of bodies blanketed under our tent, trying to sleep as best we could, knowing there was a tough day ahead.

After a truly terrible night's sleep (fortunately a search for a missing sock, feared to have been blown into the desert, was found in a sleeping bag), the four of us made our way to the start to begin the infamous long stage.

I was back in that strange head space at the beginning of the distance, knowing you are about to do something very difficult, but that you have chosen to do it. There was a slightly nervous air at the start line. People were tired from the previous night – hardly anyone had slept well in the storm – and they wanted to just get going, to start to get the miles ticked off.

We headed out. The Sahara now so very familiar to us, yet still no easier.

We passed the miles by chatting to each other, one or other of us stepping up to encourage or lead when another was flagging. We all had moments of not feeling great, of letting fatigue seep into our spirits, yet as a small group we were more robust and capable.

People were recognising us as a group who were tackling and taking on the race together.

'Here comes the cavalcade!' someone remarked as we passed in formation.

••••

Dusk changed the colour of the sky. We stood on top of a high dune, taking a moment to take in the view, looking ahead to where we were headed. There was nothing but dunes as far as we could see. We were hungry and had vowed to try not to stop before nightfall, allowing ourselves a longer checkpoint break only then.

Sophie took a swig of water.

'It's about six hours in that direction,' Tim said factually, pointing at the horizon.

'Oh good god,' groaned Sophie, saying what we were all thinking.

Six more hours seemed like another whole day's worth of energy, and almost impossible to muster.

Onwards we went, trying to maintain a determined step, just to get to the next checkpoint.

Time passed; miles passed. When we finally reached the checkpoint, we were all exhausted and took a longer stop to get some calories.

'I'm in Hell. This is Hell.' Sophie was not alone in her observation. The long stage was doing exactly what is expected of it, wringing us dry, testing us.

We became quiet as we settled in to a more rhythmic step, taking it in turns to be at the front of the four, setting the pace. Two at the front, two at the back in our now-familiar formation. The wind was picking up again, yet the air felt humid, close. Grit was swirling around in the night air as we made progress, eyes keenly focused into the dark night skies and looking for the faintest glow of the white arch of Camp.

If you keep moving, the finish comes. It always does, eventually.

With more relief than elation we made it through the long stage. Once again on this, my fourth time here, it had been done in one go, giving us a whole day's rest.

••••

The marathon stage started in another swirling sandstorm. Visibility was just about bearable, and with bandana masks wrapped around our faces we headed out, buffered and battered by the grainy swirling air. It was like sandpaper on your skin; my lips were sore, cracked and dry from the sun. As we filed out under the white arch once again, the helicopter swooped low, stirring up more sand.

This was the stage that would take us to our medals. At the start line spirits were high; we had made it this far! With the sun obscured by clouds, we had not been quite as hot, but the sandstorms had made the race gruelling. Running into a direct headwind with your feet wading through sand after a week of starving yourself is very hard work. Mercifully, after a time the wind died down and the sun began to rise with the temperatures. Sophie and I unmasked our faces and grinned at each other: *We're doing it! We're running the marathon stage in the Marathon des Sables!*

It is incredible how much energy you can muster when you feel good about yourself. The marathon miles seemed easier than any in the previous four days despite our blistered sore feet. With just three miles to go, Sophie and I shared our usual countdown, which we say to each other regardless of the race.

'Just a parkrun to go!'

We picked up our pace, legs feeling lighter with a renewed energy, knowing we had practically done it.

The cavalcade charged together in unison, all four of us egging each other on, running those last miles faster than any miles we had run all week. We were all smiles, banter and high spirits.

As the finish line approached, we instinctively held hands and formed a line, arms raised above our heads, big wide smiles of joy.

We finished the race exactly how we started it, exactly how we had started and finished each single day that week – together, a team.

••••

Several drinks in we partied back in the hotel in Ouarzazate. A tent load of female rowers were giving us a run for our money on the drinks and who could stay out the longest that night. Sharing our stories, wearing our medals, Oli and Tim D providing relentless jokes, we reminisced and laughed until our sides ached. It was truly a celebratory night to remember – and we celebrated hard!

Could we have each run that race alone? Of course we could, all of us had it within our capabilities. Would it have been as special? Not at all. In a stark contrast to the year before, this Marathon des Sables, my fourth, had been my favourite.

This race is not about the numbers, the miles. As ever with ultrarunning, it is the experience that you take away. The memories are the shared moments, the tough technical climbs, the weary lows, bunching up together against the sandstorms, the silent moments running in the dark, knowing your friends are just one step ahead of you, or next to you. There is a comfort knowing that you are doing these things together, knowing that we will always be able to relive the memories with each other in the future. This race is seeing friends overcome and conquer deep fears and seeing them realise their running dreams.

Sophie was utterly delighted at finishing – which filled me with a joy deeper than my feelings for myself. I had assumed I couldn't enjoy this race any more than I had done before – and yet once again it came up trumps.

A lot had passed in the last year – my friendship with Sophie deepening, new friends made, the cancer. And now this – it was nothing short of life-affirming. As we made our way back from the bar, laughing like school kids into the warm Sahara night, I felt so very alive – alive and happy.

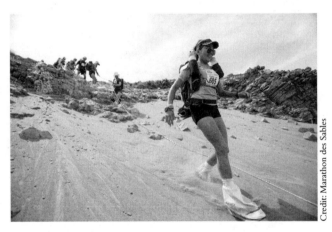

Marathon des Sables, 2018. Down the jebel.

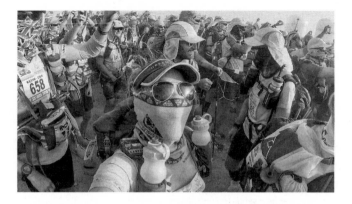

The calm after the (sand)storm. The final day's start line.

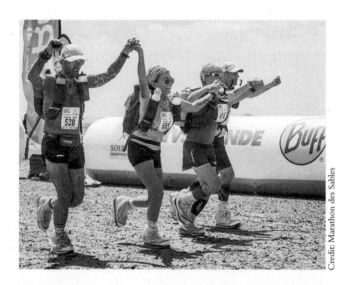

Credit: Marathon des Sables

Here comes the cavalcade!
The finish line with Sophie, Shaun and Tim D.

12

CREW LIFE

The South Downs, Grand Union Canal, Death Valley

'All I can think about is getting into the canal.
Shall I get in?'

What the hell was that? I blink hard. *Focus. Maybe eat something. Have more caffeine, that will definitely help.*

I start the engine again, reset the odometer, switch off the hazard lights and pull out into the road. Beads of sweat are trickling down my temples and I swear the shadows are taking human form. I concentrate very hard on my driving and keeping an eye out for my runner. I pass him half a mile away and keep driving for another half a mile or so and pull over.

The air is hot and heavy. Breathing it in is like inhaling hot air from a hairdryer; sickly and unpleasantly warm. Filling your lungs feels like work. The night sky is the blackest of blacks, pierced only by a sea of stars above. Here, for the first time in my life, I am in Death Valley. It is 2 a.m. and this is the second night on no sleep at all. Ahead of me the road stretches out way past the headlights of the car; there are twinkling lights of hazard indicators and runners stretched out for miles and miles. I am tired, exhausted and hungry, but this means nothing. The last thing I am here for is myself. This is crew life and the first rule of crew life is: it's all about your runner. Whatever you are going through, you must not draw attention to it, dwell on it or, heaven forbid, vocalise it. All you are here to do is to get your runner to the finish line. That is the only rule and the bottom line.

My first experience crewing and pacing was for my friend Glenn, in the South Downs Way 100, a 100-mile event. It was a long night and at times very tough for him, but watching him run around the 400-metre track at the end and going under the finish arch hit me in a way that finishing a race myself had never done. A little tear of joy for him dripped down my cheek.

Sometimes, deep into my own races, just thinking about the finish line can trigger a wobbly bottom lip, but every time I have crossed the finish line myself, it has never felt hugely emotional. Perhaps it is the tiredness; by the end of the race the emotions have been depleted, wrung out of me. Watching someone you have crewed cross the finish line can be quite a moving moment and is always a relief. For a start, you have not run the full race so are always less exhausted than they are. Then seeing what they go through, and watching them dig really deep to get their medal, is a privilege – and it is a privilege to be asked and trusted to help them do it.

••••

There is a race along the Grand Union Canal that is a non-stop 145 miles. It starts off in Gas Street in Birmingham and follows the canal tow path as it wiggles its way south through the heart of England, finally finishing in Little Venice in London. I have crewed this race three times. The first time was with my other 2013 Marathon des Sables friend, Warwick. He is a beast of a runner, fast, committed and seemingly unstoppable. This was only my second attempt at crewing and knowing that Warwick would be jostling among the top runners meant I had to make no mistakes, but keep him moving as best I possibly could.

He was over 110 miles in when I joined him for the last stint and he was still running well. At least, he looked like he was running well. We continued along the canal at a respectable run pace for the distance. Warwick was fixated on the point where we passed the M25, which meant for him the home straight. In this race, the home straight was around a marathon still to go.

We stopped at one of the checkpoints, which are really strung out in a race this length. Aware that Warwick had not eaten anything for a couple of hours, I tried him with one of the freshly cooked bacon sandwiches put together by the friendly checkpoint staff. He took one bite and almost immediately threw up what was clearly more than a single bite of food. No more bacon sandwiches, then. After that he made it all the way to the end, 25 miles, sucking on just three Haribo sweets. It was not the first or last time I would witness an ultrarunner defying medical science and being able to continue to run many miles on no calories whatsoever.

You would think that following a canal is straightforward – and generally it is, though also mind-numbingly monotonous. Just make sure you stay next to the water; how hard can it be?

Well, there are times when you have to cross over a bridge to pick up the right towpath, and each bridge has a number. We had information about the bridges to cross and this fell to me, and not just because I was the pacer and crew: I had not already run 112 miles, so my brain was obviously sharper.

It should not have been confusing, even if the bridges weren't always sequential: some have been replaced over time or an extra bridge has been added and given the label A, B or even C. Any wrong turn would, of course, mean extra steps for Warwick.

I made a mistake early on, taking him over a bridge which forced him to double back.

Thankfully that was a short learning curve for me and not repeated.

I went on to pace this race twice more. Emily Foy was next. We met while running around Anglesey, had completed several marathons together and she helped me greatly in the 2015 Marathon des Sables in the Sahara Desert. She is simply another remarkable runner. Endlessly polite and charming, yet with a quiet and steely determination, she is one of the toughest ultrarunners I know. She was trucking along at a reasonable pace and being her usual affable self. We were around 120 miles in when she said she was feeling hot and that her heart rate was too high: 'All I can think about is getting into the canal. Shall I get in?'

I eyeballed the murky water. The top of the water had thin, suspicious, brown sludgy puddles and greasy oil spots. There was a carrier bag and old SKOL beer can and lots of cigarettes butts floating in it. 'That's not a great idea, Emily.'

'Just my legs, then. Or arms. I just want to cool down.'

It's not particularly warm at all. 'How about a drink?'

'I really would like a pint of lager.'

This was the last thing I expected her to request. I thought perhaps a can of Coke or even a cup of tea.

'Maybe a pub will be open soon! There's a few along the route.'

I googled and with a stroke of luck we would indeed arrive at a pub after a few miles. It's late morning and the pub had only just opened, but I ran in and asked for a shandy. 'Only a tiny little bit of lager please, mainly lemonade.'

This was not what Emily requested, but I thought a full pint after 130 miles might not be the best idea.

She drank it practically in one go and got running again.

She was moving very well, but still said she didn't feel right and that her heart rate was too high. I didn't give this too much thought and put it down to the huge distance she had run.

It didn't slow her down at all and she crossed the line after 145 miles, delighted to be the woman in second place. I was exhausted and looked dishevelled. She changed her clothes and brushed her hair, and looked fresh as the morning, chatting convivially to all there.

Not long after, I got a text message from her explaining why her heart rate had been so high. She was pregnant! Several months later, she delivered a happy and healthy baby boy. Remarkable.

••••

Cat Simpson is someone I have known from one of my first ever ultramarathons. There was a brief period of time back then when we managed the same speed. For a couple of races we ran together, pushing each other on. Some of my fastest times date from when I was as fast as Cat. Her true calibre emerged not long after. She would go on to earn a GB vest and represent the country at ultrarunning, while I would stay in the middle of the pack.

I crewed her for the last leg of the 145 miles along the Grand Union Canal. My alarm went off in the middle of the night and the 30+ miles I was supposed to be running had already been seriously curtailed by Cat going astonishingly fast, burning through the miles at record pace. Leaping into my car, I drove to the next agreed meeting point.

Standing on the now-familiar towpath, I arrived just in time to see her running towards me. I was with her dad, Keith, a great runner himself. She looked fluid, light on her feet, effortless – it was impressive. However, as soon as she stopped, she looked wobbly on her feet, unsteady. It seemed to take her a moment to recognise me. After a few seconds of just staring at me, she said, 'I thought you were a post.'

Running a long time can make you see things strangely.

She ate a snack, still looking unsteady. She knew she was on for a great time and seconds after she had swallowed her food began running again. As soon as she broke into a run, she looked great again, light and fluid. It was both baffling and brilliant to witness.

'You're just going to have to stay running!' her smiling dad called after her as she ran off down the narrow towpath.

We both waited for her at the finish and saw her coming around the corner to finish, triumphantly. She completed the course in a staggering 27 hours, setting a new course record and propelling herself into the world of elite ultrarunning. Winners get a brightly painted pot, decorated like traditional Narrowboat Bargeware. It was very jolly, and Cat clutched on to it as her dad and I practically carried her to my car from the finish line. I drove them both back; she was half asleep but still tried to make polite conversation. Thankfully, both were so very tired they did not realise I looped round the Hanger Lane gyratory three times before I finally got myself in the correct lane; I too was rather tired.

••••

Up there with races I have crewed and paced as much as the Grand Union Canal are Centurion-branded races. Notably, Autumn 100: it seems that I am there almost every year, running along the lonely cold fields, into the misty riverside paths, steering people in on the last 25 miles. One time it was so cold the water in my bottles froze. A couple of times I've been there to bring home friends who did not quite get the time they wanted. It's a great race – perfectly pitched with not too much elevation, but just enough to make it interesting. It's also the home of my own 100-mile personal best.

On one very cold night I did something memorably embarrassing. Every single time I go back to Goring Village Hall, the race epicentre and hub, someone on the race staff will recount the story to me or assembled guests and laugh.

You arrive in the middle of the night to pace the last leg – anything from midnight to 3 a.m., depending on how fast your runner is. I opted not to sleep and headed there to wait in the hall overnight, soaking up the atmosphere, seeing friends and generally trying not to get under anyone's feet.

It was about midnight and I parked my car in a side road and walked over to the hall. I said my hellos and asked if anyone needed any help with anything.

I was waiting patiently when two police officers walked in. It was the middle of the night in the middle of peaceful, rural Oxfordshire. The officers gazed around, taking in the faces, and Nici Griffin, in charge of the space, approached them, asking if she could be of any help. There were heads nodding, murmurs, and she glanced my way. More nodding.

'Susie, can we have a word?'

Jesus CHRIST! What has happened? My mind immediately flashed to my daughter. *Is she OK? Is everything OK?*

'Miss Chan?'

'Yes.'

'Are you the owner of a red Ford Ka?'

'Yes.'

'Are you aware it's currently in the front garden of a dwelling around the corner?'

'It's what?' I had left the car parked safely. How could this have happened?

Easily, really, if you leave the handbrake off. After I walked off, it rolled down a hill, miraculously avoided crashing into any other vehicles and careered into a garden. The house owners, not surprisingly rather alarmed at seeing a random car appear in the middle of the night squashing their roses, had called the police.

The quick detective work from this point was impressive. A registration check led them to my house in the dead of night. No answer. Next, they googled me and saw that I was an ultrarunner. Aware of the local race, they put two and two together. They were jolly decent about it all and after giving me a ticking-off, posed for a picture with me, my cheeks burning red with embarrassment.

Now every year when I go back to crew the A100 race, I am reminded of the time my car nearly caused havoc in the sleepy village and repeatedly asked if I have left the handbrake on.

I have a soft spot for that race. The last section is the same path that takes in the endless field and gate section of the Thames Path 100, my first 100-mile effort. The end of these races can vary so much from person to person and you see it all close up when crewing. I have crewed my friend Scott there, an accomplished runner who takes on 200-mile races (yes, they are a thing!). He was so fast at the end I had to pull out some seriously fast miles to keep up. I also crewed my friend Mike, who had to make a Herculean effort during those last, never-ending miles through the fields. A tough and experienced runner, he was having a very bad day at the end, toughing it out while riding the rollercoaster of emotions that went from laughing to silent tears back to laughing in the space of a single field; the sort of behaviour that only pushing yourself to your physical edge can produce.

••••

Crew and pacers are not compulsory in a lot of UK races, but are in many others, especially races in the US. No one has ever been a DNF (Did Not Finish) under my watch, but we came perilously close one year when I was crewing Iwan Thomas on his first attempt at 100 miles.

Iwan is an athletics World Champion, an Olympian; he knows how to run, it's in his blood. The only problem is he is used to running for 400 metres. One hundred miles is over 400 times 400 metres. Everything he ever had to learn about running, he had to unlearn. This was not about speed and power, this was about slow, steady and controlled running.

His training in the lead-up had been anything but ideal. A combination of lockdown and his own reluctance to get out for solo long runs added to the lack of consistency. We covered miles and miles, and climbed so many hills together in training, that a strong friendship was formed. Yet as the date of the race approached, it became apparent that it would be touch and go for him even to make the start line.

All runners had to run a qualifying 50-mile run, Olympian or not. Iwan was not keen on it, with a valid concern that he would run the 50 and then realise just how difficult 100 miles would be. Lockdown was cancelling races so in the end we had to make do with just creating a route and running 50 miles. After procrastination and then firm commitment on Iwan's part, just in the nick of time he pulled an accomplished 50-mile qualifying time out of the bag. It was game on.

The day started promisingly. They were off! The great British summertime had pulled a blinder and it was over 25°C. Lovely for a sit-down in the back garden with a cold drink, less so for 100 miles of the South Downs Way. The trail is exposed in many parts, meaning you are out in direct sunlight for most of the course. As the day progressed, the heat was taking its toll on the runners. Iwan deliberately slowed in the heat of the day, keeping his heart rate low and spirits up. It was not until dusk when things unravelled.

First, there was a stressful call from home. His son had to be taken into hospital as an emergency. Iwan's partner told me that there would be nothing he could do: COVID rules meant he would not be allowed in the building, so he should stay out running and she would keep us posted.

After a few agonising minutes, Iwan weighed everything up and kept moving forward, his worry now eating away at his energy.

After a while we came into a checkpoint and the staff in the space immediately started to rush us on. There was a rolling start to the race and we had miscalculated just how close Iwan now was to the cut-off: 'You have seven minutes to get out of here!'

The cut-off means automatic withdrawal from the race. We had to get out quickly. Seven minutes in a race of 100 miles is virtually nothing – a time that could be easily lost on one tough hill, one loo break or one checkpoint. I suddenly thought that we would not make it: he still had so far to go, and some of the biggest hills of the course and the draining overnight section were still to come.

With everything to lose, the only thing left to do was to put in a charge.

What I saw Iwan do from that moment on was nothing short of incredible. I witnessed the essence of what it takes to make someone rise up to be an Olympian, the fighting spirit you need just to keep pushing, to keep attacking when everything hurts and your brain is telling you to stop. Pushing against the odds, the poor training, the toughness of the night section, the mental and physical challenges of running 100 miles, the worry about his son.

There was no way he was going to fail. He was not prepared to let that happen. Every minute and every step from that moment forward was counted, pushed, focused. He was unrelenting in his mental attitude. Watching him in this intense state targeting the finish, I realised he would not fail. The last miles were hilly, arduous, exhausting. The sun had risen again and was beginning to beat down upon us, and still Iwan kept one foot in front of the other, never losing pace or letting his resolve slacken.

Around 800 metres from the finish, I called out, 'It's done. You've done it, Iwan!'

'No. Not until the finish line. Anything could happen still. I might not make it. Will I make it?'

We came from completely different backgrounds in running, yet here we were together in this race. In these last few steps before he reached the finish line, that former Olympian refused to take success for granted.

Watching him make that final lap, the slowest 400 metres of his life, was emotional, nothing short of heart-warming. He had made it – and he had made it happen.

••••

You don't have to be at the front to be the greatest. In ultrarunning the ones at the back are the ones on their feet the longest. The ones who have had to tough it out mentally for hours more than anyone else. All of the things that make ultrarunning difficult have to be suffered for the most time for those at the back. Everyone, from the runner in first to those in the middle to those at the end, has their own challenges, difficulties to overcome and moments of glory. Everyone has travelled the same distance, achieved the same feat.

Sometimes when you are running the races yourself, these moments are lost on you; in a blur of fatigue and focus you can miss moments, not take in the details. Crewing and pacing offers the opportunity to be right at the heart of the race and the ability to see it through a different perspective. Any race is about the people you meet, the things you learn, and crewing lets you give back to the community.

You are rewarded not by the finish, but very much by the journey.

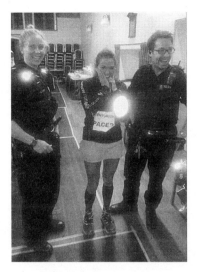

Can you get arrested for leaving the handbrake off?
Full of embarrassment with police officers while crewing the
Autumn 100 in Oxfordshire.

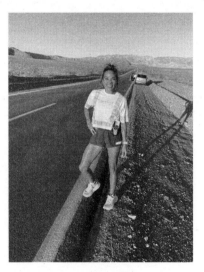

The first rule of crew life: it's all about your runner.
Sunrise in Death Valley.

13

I AM A RUNNER

2019

'My wardrobe of dresses, jeans, heels had given way to race T-shirts, running shorts, trainers.'

I stand at the top of the stairs contemplating the best descent.

One step at a time, sideways? Let's try that.

My body aches. I've not just run a tough marathon, or been training extremely hard. It's just another day in the week for me. I assume this is just how it is now.

It must be my age, I tell myself as I make my way down. 'Things just fall off a cliff when you get past 40, Susie,' my mother used to say.

Not for the first time I marvel at how we take for granted how easily we move about when we're in our teens and twenties. Your body works alongside you much more when you are young. My face left a dent in the bedsheets back then, not the other way round like it does now. I rub the crease the pillow has left on my cheek.

The good news is, the aches will ease a bit if I keep moving about and then I'll be walking up and down the stairs normally in an hour. *First, a cup of tea.*

••••

There have been so many little things that seem to slow me down a little more now. At 45, I'm not exactly old. I will walk into a room with a strong sense of urgency, only to find myself standing there, wondering what on earth it could be that I need from this room. Words escape me.

'Pass me the . . . thing . . . the . . . you know.' Pointing and miming actions do their best to fill in the lack of words. I live in a perpetual state of never knowing where my front door keys are.

And running is harder, sweatier, slower. Trail runs are now plods through the mud. A couple of years ago, I relished the terrain, bouncing around from one foot to the other, the slippery mud gathering in the tread of my trainers, and running fast through puddles, the sludgy water splashing up my legs, for the sheer thrill. Paced road running is now noticeably lacklustre. Maybe I have run too much? I get out most days and usually it's all fine really, just ticking along. It's speed that eludes me. A few attempts at fast running back at the track, sessions I used to love, leave me breathless and dripping in salty sweat, with little niggles in my calves and way off pace.

I have just emerged from a couple of years of thyroid problems, which affected my overall fitness, and this is a new phase of life. One where running is slow, one where I simply cannot remember what an envelope is called, one where first thing in the morning I am as creaky as the stairs.

••••

A couple of years before this, in 2017, when I had no idea my own thyroid was doing its very best to work against me, I went through a phase when running ended up making me feel sad. I lost the joy.

The thing about running is this: when you are new to it and are relatively consistent about training, it is a succession of improvements. Your whole first year of running is about setting personal bests. This is when you learn how to pace yourself and fuel yourself, strengthening your results. As you gain experience, your confidence grows. The two things become intertwined, symbiotic. It was simple: when I ran well, I felt good about myself.

For the first few years as a runner, I could just turn up to a 10K, a half-marathon or marathon and bust out a respectable time that was pretty consistent. There were a few injuries here and there, typical when you are new to running, but you learn, you recover and you build back. Afterwards I was able just to slot back into races at the same pace. It came so easily. I found myself reflecting on those happy days and realised how much I took them for granted.

Then I became unwell. Not enough to raise a red flag, not enough to think something was seriously wrong, but enough to leave me tired, breathless and hungry all the time.

Probably the ultra training, my head told me.

There were other things that, though I did not know, were showcase symptoms of a thyroid problem. I got heavier, I could not breathe so well. What used to be my steady run pace became harder and harder to achieve.

I'd head out for my run and push myself to get anything near my usual pace. And it was agony, feeling like I was running flat out, my heart pumping hard against my ribs, air restricted and tight in my throat. All just to run half a mile at what used to be a comfortable pace. I looked back at some of my race results, achieved with ease, and wished I had applied myself better, feeling like there were opportunities missed. Sometimes when looking back at race results today, I can never really understand how it was at all possible.

I was by no means super-fast, never bothering the front of races, but by my own standards the times and results were enough for me to be pleased and they were consistent.

Back then as my pace began to dwindle, so did my joy for running. Trying and trying to be faster, I became frustrated, annoyed. I started to make excuses not to meet people to run, not wanting to be the one who was always trying to catch up at the back, or the slowest, the sweatiest. I was afraid of people looking at my pace on my uploads to Strava and judging. Running went from being something that brought me happiness to one that made me stressed about pacing, or feeling disappointed.

Even so, I did not stop running. I kept on going out, kept on moving, mainly solo so I could suffer it alone. The habit of running was too much to stop. I have often described my relationship with running as being rather akin to a religion. Once I found it, it became more than a hobby, it became part of who I am, a deeply ingrained part of my life. It was not all-consuming, but it was something which I thought about or did almost every day, part of the fabric of me. I am a runner.

My circle of friends had slowly shifted from ones who met up for a beer on a Friday night to ones who met up for a trail run on a Sunday morning. My wardrobe of dresses, jeans, heels had given way to race T-shirts, running shorts, trainers.

Over time, I slowly slid into a more pedestrian pace. I still made myself go out running, sometimes reluctantly, sometimes with dread, sometimes with hours between the decision to head out for the run and the action itself, but I did always get out. It was difficult.

The acceptance that I was slowing down was not gradual or even easy. It took more of a committed effort. I still wanted to run, I wanted to run fast, but I could not run as fast any more. Plodding along by myself on the trails gave me time to think.

Why is this bothering me? Running is better when it makes you happy. So why am I hanging all my happiness on how fast I can run?

For a mixture of reasons: a little bit of ego, a dollop of insecurity, a worry about my ageing. All things within my own head.

I unpicked these one at a time. *Are people scrutinising my Strava and remarking at how pedestrian I have become? Probably not. And if they are, that might be a reflection on their own relationship with running, which is not something I can control.*

I asked myself, *Do I really care what some random person thinks of my pace? After all, it's my running and not theirs.*

I scrolled through a couple of elite ultrarunners I follow, saw that a few of them posted lots of slow-paced runs. It was actually quite comforting. People you admire just out for an easy run. No classic Strava behaviour where the excuses are all piled into the title to explain away the pace – these are recovery runs and only a few seconds a mile slower anyway, or the run partners are the problem, or the weather, or anything. No, just some slow, plodding runs.

It dawned on me that they were setting a great example. People do not ultimately care about your pace; they care only about their own. You are simply a benchmark against their own fitness. Something to aim for, to beat, or to compare yourself with, something to look at and realise that it's possible to run at a variety of intensities, driven by different reasons.

Among my own friends there is genuine happiness when we do well and very simply no judgement if we do not. That's how it should be. *Do I really care what other people think about my running?*

A little bit, yes.

But do I want to hang my own relationship with this thing I love on other people's opinions?

No.

I came to the conclusion that if I want to push myself in a run, and am trying as hard as I can, then there simply is nothing more to do.

Letting it go was now easy – and letting go of what people think of you is one of the most liberating things you can do. It felt very good indeed.

I reframed my attitude and set about doing a few things to help me find my enjoyment again.

I decided not to worry about the digits on my watch. Heading out for runs, I turned my watch inwards on my wrist so I could not to see the pace. (Heaven forbid I did not record a run, though. I wasn't going to go cold turkey.)

I got back out there again, making the purpose of my runs to meet my friends, socialise and catch up on their lives.

If running alone, I made the goal to head out to a specific destination, something as simple as seeing where a new trail leads, or somewhere that offered a pretty photo I could take, or somewhere new to explore.

The focus was firmly set on the experience rather than the pace.

My running reignited back to joy.

••••

OK, running slower no longer bothered me, but the feeling of creaky joints did. *Is this the rest of my life now?*

In late 2019 I was running one day with Jane, a friend from my local running club, when she said something to me which changed everything: 'Sounds like you are perimenopausal!'

It had not occurred to me. Why not? Though I was 45 years old, I assumed the symptoms related to my compromised thyroid. Functioning on a third of a thyroid gland, I just thought all my issues were somehow connected to that. Instinctively knowing something was off-kilter but not knowing what, I kept returning again and again to my doctor, getting him to check and double-check my thyroid. On the last visit he gently told me, 'You are allowed to have other things wrong with you.'

The list of perimenopausal symptoms are broad and vary from person to person. Piecing them all together, I realised Jane was right. Just because I was not breaking out in hot flushes did not mean I was not going through the menopause. The aching joints were my most painful symptom; some days I had to take painkillers to get a reasonable night's sleep. Other symptoms ranged from annoying – tinnitus, spots, strange itches that travelled all over my body, hair sprouting forth on my face while thinning on my head – to ones which were more troubling – night-time anxiety, staring into the night and stressing about the most minute things. There were long periods of lethargy, and at times a crippling and embarrassing forgetfulness.

It was a comfort to finally figure this out. At the time getting a prescription for hormone replacement therapy (HRT) was difficult because the UK was in lockdown, but eventually I got over that hurdle and within days I started to feel better. The aches did not quite go away but subsided considerably. Other symptoms practically disappeared. I embarked on more mobility exercises, some gentle and targeted strength training, and started practising yoga again. Yoga was something I had enjoyed in the past, but this time I threw myself into it, from more dynamic yoga to some restorative relaxing sessions.

Within weeks I felt different, better, younger!

One day I was halfway down the stairs when I noticed I was descending them one at a time, normally. No aches, no sideways walking. Relief.

This is getting older, an inevitable next stage of life and something I am embracing. I might be slower, yet I see some of my friends who are going through the menopause, or who are out the other side, and they are running personal bests, fast marathons, still chasing the pace. Will that be me? Probably not, because this is not a huge driver for me anymore, but it's good to know there's always light at the end of the tunnel; that you can still choose to chase pace as an older woman if you have the desire; that you can still run if you want to.

There are moments when the symptoms and the aches return. It comes in waves, and some days are harder, but some days I feel like the old me. On the days when it's worse, things feel more like a test physically. My memory remains appalling. I look in the mirror and see a new addition to an increasingly hairy chin, a thinner hairline, a wrinkle deepening – but then I remember I can still run 100 miles and that there is still joy in my running.

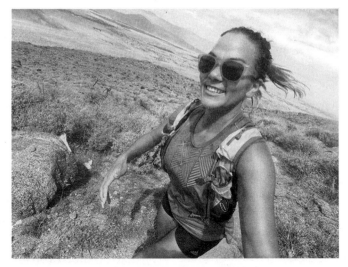

Enjoying the trails in the Anza-Borrego desert in southern California.

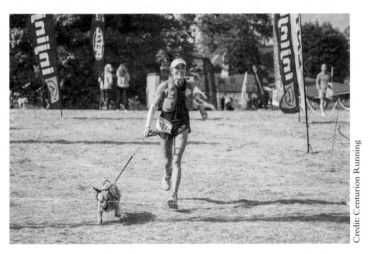

Finishing the North Downs Way 50 – my dog Manny joined me for the last 100 metres.

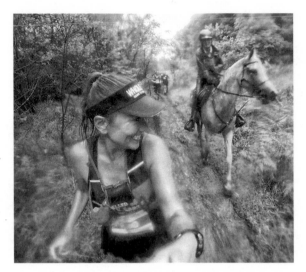

Man v horse in Llanwrtyd Wells, Wales.
One of my favourite races in the world.

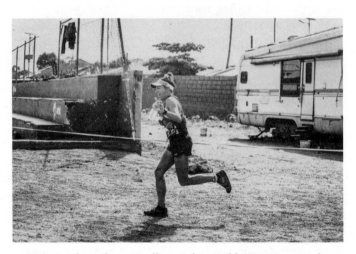

Running has taken me all over the world. Here I am at the
Sierra Leone Marathon in 2019.

14
HUNDREDS OF MILES
OF NOTHINGNESS

Badwater, 2023

'It's not Badwater unless you suffer, Susie.'

I stare up the road, which stretches out in a perfect straight line for miles and miles into the heat haze of the horizon. I narrow my eyes to try to follow it as it hits the foothills of the mountains and then disappears up, up and up, hugging the curves of the ascent.

It's blisteringly, oppressively hot.

I look down at the brakes of the car; we all do. They are smoking and the smell of melting rubber fills our noses.

'A few more minutes and they should be good to go!' Chris Howe nods encouragingly in his upbeat way.

This is not a great situation. The brakes have overheated driving down a mountain descent 17 miles long. Our hired automatic car has no downshift or gear options, so we have pulled over to avoid brake failure. We cannot stand around for too long, though: we are in the hottest place on Earth, Death Valley. The average life expectancy here without water is just 14 hours. Fortunately, we have a couple of bottles each, and occasionally a car passes. I suspect they are doing what we are doing: checking out the race route for Badwater 135, the race

I have had my heart set on for the entire time I have known about ultrarunning.

I am quiet, thinking about all the ways the car could fail now – and if the car fails, I am out of the race. You need the vehicle to survive. I have trained so hard for this race, months of running along puddle-soaked trails in the pouring rain, on treadmills in heat chambers, accumulating hundreds of miles in my legs and adapting my body to prepare for the severe heat. I cannot imagine a worse way to be out of the race than car failure; I would rather break a bone. As I am thinking about this and staring up the road, my crew are huddling round the other side of the vehicle.

Chris has spotted a nail coming out of the tyre. In a silent nod of agreement, my crew – Chris, Shaun, Phil and Debbie – collectively and wordlessly agree that it is best not to let me know.

I am unaware as we get back into the car and drive on with the nail still in place to Badwater Basin, a barren salt plain which will be the race start.

•••

It is 4 July and everything apart from a couple of restaurants and one shop is closed. Lone Pine is a tiny town on the edge of the Mojave Desert with the stunning backdrop of the Sierra Nevada mountain range. This is Wild West Country, with wagon wheels and saloon doors, and it is absolutely roasting hot here.

Shaun disappeared for a couple of hours and now has arrived back with a variety of things purchased from the garage. 'Just in case we get a puncture!' I am so engrossed in my own thoughts, my own mental preparation and faffing with the huge amount of race kit I have brought that it does not occur to me that this was for a possible puncture, rather than my crew being extra cautious.

My crew are perfect company, neither too exuberant and excitable nor too laid-back and unbothered. We head out for food and some beers, just being around them makes me feel comfortable and safe; our banter is relaxed. As well as Shaun, who is well versed in dealing with me in ultrarunning situations, I have Chris Howe from my heat training days and world record treadmill run, who has now earned a PhD in ultrarunning. He is Dr Ultrarunning!

I am delighted that Debbie Martin-Consani, one of the UK's most prolific, established and respected ultrarunners, is joining the crew. Having represented Team GB, she is a safe pair of hands. I crewed for her in this very race last year and she is now repaying the favour.

Lastly, there is Phil Hill, photographer and videographer friend, who is very genial, has crewed for me previously in a race called Salton Sea (another Badwater race) and can seemingly survive with virtually no sleep. This is a very useful skill, because these four people will be staying together for two nights and up to two days, sitting in a car with virtually no sleep and only periodic air conditioning. It's a tough gig.

Each person brings their own skill set. Chris, Crew Chief, is organised and gentle, and he understands the physiology of the body under the impact of heat and ultrarunning combined. He approaches everything with an organised demeanour that only a scientist can and he creates spreadsheets for fun. Shaun is my emotional buffer, for times when I am feeling weak and want to have a little secret cry, and is also likely to help me in any undignified loo-stop moments when my quads do not work. Phil is a workhorse, thoughtful, easy-going and – very importantly to me in this social media world – takes great photos. I want these because I plan on doing this only once and want decent pictures to post and to have as a memory.

Debbie, who has broken course records and won some of the most gnarly ultramarathons, gave the most impressively gritty performance on this course last year. For more than 100 miles, she was throwing up. I have never seen anyone move forward in such a steadfast and determined way on virtually no calories. She showed no signs whatsoever of weakness at any moment, just cracked on with it – the very definition of badass. She was the one who finally convinced me to do it. The most important thing about having Debbie on the crew is that I do not at any moment want to look pathetic in front of her; she's like the cool kid in the playground I want to impress, and I want to show off in front of her, to show her that I am capable. That may seem slightly juvenile, but I need the attitude; this race is notoriously difficult.

'What is the most difficult race you have run, Debbie?'

She ponders for a moment. 'This one.'

Really? Out of all of them?

'People might go to Chamonix for a trail run, or run in the mountains, but who says, "I'll just pop to Death Valley for a run"? No one.'

••••

You cannot simply enter this race; you need to be invited. Ideally you will have a robust CV of race finishes and the race organisers also like you to have experienced the course either as crew or volunteering. This makes perfect sense as they want you to have seen the route in the hottest time of year when the event takes place; to have felt what it is like to have that heat on your skin and the remoteness.

Years ago, when I heard about this race, I said: 'I love deserts, I want to do it.' And I did want to do it, I really did. I thought it sounded great. The thing about Badwater 135, though, is this: reading about it, or looking at photos of it, does not do the race justice at all. You simply cannot get the race from images or words. This is a race that needs to be seen and felt to be believed.

So, saying that I wanted to do the race without having any experience, and having only ever known the heat of the Sahara in April, was rather like saying I wanted to climb Everest – not impossible but a bit of a leap. This is an extremely difficult race, one in a league of its own. Yes, you can dream – and dream I did. Subsequently I found out that more people have actually climbed Everest than finished this race. Five times more people, in fact, have got to the top of the highest mountain in the world than have got their hands on the finisher's buckle of Badwater 135. Just getting to the start line was a challenge; getting that golden ticket became my long-term goal.

I spent 12 years running, learning, gathering experiences. I honed my heat experience in multiple desert races and took myself to races in humid jungles, sweltering in Peru and Costa Rica, and back to the Sahara. Over the years I accumulated the failures of several attempts at trying to get my nutrition right; nutrition is always my downfall, and over and over again I battled nausea and deep fatigue to get to finish lines while testing it out, seeing whether that was palatable (Pot Noodles seem to be the pinnacle of my ultramarathon nutrition game). I spent agonising hours toughening my battered feet by running 100-mile races on roads rather than trails, some of these races consisting of virtually no turns, just 100 miles of straight road stretching out in front of you until fading to a dot on the horizon, seemingly never-ending, the repetitive step after step after step on the tarmac making my feet swell and my bones hurt.

I have run around and around in circles on a track in the pouring rain, listening to a godawful piccolo; run on a treadmill for 12 hours with only a bucket for a loo; run through marathon finish lines in cities I would never otherwise have seen; hallucinated while trying not to fall into a river. I have hated running, loved it, hated it all over again, been intimidated, excited and scared by it. It has consumed me, bored me, thrilled me, humiliated me – and lifted me up higher than I ever thought or dreamed possible. It has given me life.

There have been thousands and thousands of miles of running. In my Peloton classes I coach people to their own personal goals, whether training for their own ultramarathon or their first time running a mile, and I often say: 'You never regret a run.' As I look back on all the things I have done, I do not regret a single one, even the ones where I have fallen over.

Running slowly overtook my life. When I started, I was working in a museum, and now I had somehow turned running into a career. It was not by design or ambition; it came about organically. I began to document my journey, keeping it honest and positive. I used social media as the space to share stories and run selfies and to connect with fellow runners. I can imagine there are heaps of people out there who quite frankly are not interested in my smiling selfie somewhere deep into an ultramarathon, but there were some. As my participation in ultrarunning grew, so did the popularity of the sport and the opportunities that came my way.

There was a point when I was juggling working five days a week in a full-time job trying to be a good mother, meanwhile cramming the run training around those two things. I did not think life could be any other way until little job offers trickled in. Brands wanted me to try their new trainers, invited me to events, then I got asked to be on podcasts, interviewed in magazines, and then one day I got an offer of sponsorship. It took a lot of courage on my part to take the leap of faith to resign from my steady job, to forgo the monthly salary, to go it alone. All I had ever known was a monthly pay cheque, set days off. The sponsorship was just enough to get by, anything else would be a bonus, I told myself. I was commentating at races, working with brands, hosting events like the National Running Show, and then one day out of the blue in 2020 Peloton messaged me. They were launching their treadmill in the UK and would like a chat. Initially I thought they wanted me to take one for a few months, share what it was like on social media, much like the other opportunities I had.

'We are looking for instructors.'

Me?

Really?

'Do you know how old I am?!'

They did and they did not care about that; they wanted someone passionate about fitness, who was authentic. I auditioned and got the job as an instructor. For me, it was like landing my dream job, the pinnacle of where my running could take me. Here, I could share my love of running and my journey with it, and more importantly, encourage and join people on theirs. It was a space where we could laugh about it, talk about it, work at it. I could connect, grow and continue on my running journey with a whole new and bigger audience.

The thing about running is that it is never complete, it is never done, you have never ever learned all there is to learn about running and experienced all there is to experience. You cannot have the highs without the lows. You have to accept it will never just be a series of highs. It is what it is, this is what it is like to be a runner. Only you can decide where the journey ends.

••••

In February 2023 I got the invite I had been dreading and hoping for in equal measure: Badwater 135. By this point I had been out three times to crew, going through the same circle of emotions every time: arriving in Death Valley to crew the race, seeing exactly what it's like close up, thinking it's nothing short of absolutely fucking ridiculous, and coming home knowing it's too difficult for me. Then over time forgetting the ludicrous tiredness caused by losing two nights' sleep, the stifling unbreathable heat, the savage mountain ascents – and deciding to come back again to crew. And so the whole cycle would start again.

Three things happened in succession which made me decide to throw my name in for consideration: COVID-19 came along and all of a sudden the choices we might like to make were taken away from us, our worlds shrunk to our gardens, balconies and windows. Next, I started to be perimenopausal; my joints ached just from lying down and an easy run became like wading through treacle. Running became my yardstick to how I was feeling within myself, while also helping me. The ability to just go and run became both a mental and physical challenge while simultaneously becoming my saviour through COVID and bodily changes. There was a distinct lack of pace and it did not matter, as there were no races to train for. I fell in love with it all over again. The simplicity of being outside and moving was enough, and I was grateful for it.

Then, COVID calmed down and Debbie Martin-Consani asked me to crew for her and put in such a gritty performance, somehow making it look manageable despite all the vomit. At the end she looked at me in a knowing, wise manner and said in her very matter-of-fact way: 'You know you are going to have to do it, Susie. Just put your name in the hat.'

It was what I needed to hear, what I needed to be told, so I did – *and here we are in Death Valley.*

••••

The nearest thing I had experienced to this heat is opening an oven door to take out the roast dinner. The air hit you and breathing it in made your throat hot. The phrase *You could fry an egg on it* is often misused, but here you could literally fry an egg on the road, on your car, even on the seat of the car if you did not put a cover on it. This was dangerous, this was blisteringly hot.

I had gone through the biggest, most specific training block in my life to get here. Chris organised a rigorous heat training schedule, which I obediently suffered through, sweating up to 2 kg each hour and then going off to work in order to run again, broadcasting live globally for Peloton. I hydrated with cans of Coke, sugar and caffeine, replenishing my energy so I could in turn be the energy and the motivation for thousands of others joining in to run as a community. Towards the end of my heat training, I wore jumpers in the heat chamber, pushing my core temperature up each time, pushing the limits of what my body found manageable. It was relentless and exhausting.

I ran for hundreds of miles in the dreary British weather, battered by wind and rain. I lifted weights, I practised yoga, I spent evenings diligently doing boring physio exercises, balancing on one foot and then the other.

· I raced too: Salton Sea with my friend Emma Harris, 81 miles of desert and up a mountain – a 'mini Badwater'. It's a team event in that you have to stay together for the whole race; the only exception for not running together is to have a comfort break, and even then only a few metres are allowed or you face disqualification. I felt sick in the heat, but Emma stayed strong and pulled me through tough sections until we had done well in the race. I also ran well in the other race in the Badwater series, the 50-mile Cape Fear.

Now, if I complete Badwater 135, I will be the first European female to finish all three of the race series in a year. Not that I felt like I needed any more motivation.

••••

I thought I would be a bag of nerves at the start line. Instead, I felt calm and controlled, much like my very first Marathon des Sables. It was dusk and the mildly sulphuric smell of Badwater Basin filled the air, swirling and mixing with our feelings of anticipation. Finally, this was it.

The crew cars were all lit up with lights – each with its own distinctive colour or pattern – and crew members were excited to be part of the event. Badwater Basin sits 280 feet below sea level and is the lowest point of North America. From there we would run on road for 135 miles through the hottest and one of the most dangerous places on earth – Death Valley – where we were to traverse over three mountain ranges climbing 14,000 feet, finally making the final climb up Mount Whitney, the highest point in the contiguous United States. We had 48 hours. This is widely considered one of the gold stars and toughest events in ultrarunning.

Chris Kostman, the race director, resplendent in a cowboy hat, gathered us together. He was in his element, eyes shining bright as he made jokes at our expense and put us all at ease. This is his baby, and I have never been to a race with so much information and thought put into its organisation. He has an eye for detail, probably because he is himself an experienced endurance athlete: he was the youngest person to win Race Across America, cycling across the continent at the age of 21. He understands what it is like to put yourself through the wringer for the love of sport.

'It's not Badwater unless you suffer, Susie,' he told me as I worried in the weeks before the race, doubting my ability. One thing that was really playing on my mind was the 'cut-off' times that the race includes. Here in Death Valley, I would have 14 hours to make the 50-mile cut-off. A time which on paper is well within my ability, but in the desert things are slower. Notably, we start at night and you straight away lose a night's sleep running. All of my long races had taught me one thing: I am not great in races overnight. Having done quite well in the other two Badwater races, I had been placed in the middle wave to leave. An hour before me a large group had left already, then it would be the next wave of about 30 runners, and then after us the Elites. I would need to be very careful with pacing. Ultramarathons are the same as 5K races and any other races in this regard. If you start out too quickly, you will pay the price later. I could not go out so hard I made the 50-mile cut off, but blew up later. It was going to be hard enough as it was.

That's the thing about this race: you stand on the start line knowing full well that you are going to be in pain, that it will hurt you for hours, and that you have chosen to be here. *I know this, and right now, breathing in the hot night air, I am happy with my choice. This is where I am meant to be. There is nothing more I can do but run.*

••••

The American National Anthem played out and we counted down from 10 to one and I started running the biggest race of my life. Telling myself this would be a one-off, and no matter what agonies lay ahead I must make the headspace to try to enjoy it, to try to observe and absorb the race.

I started off with a bandana full of ice around my neck. Melting away in cooling drips, it trickled down my neck. The temperature was around 38°C, or 100°F, even though it was night-time.

I headed out of Badwater Basin on the boardwalk and out on to the tarmac road and into the first night of running. The first few miles passed uneventfully and peacefully. The pack of runners in my starting wave spread out quickly, and soon it was just the sound of our own feet on the tarmac and the strange shapes and outline of the desert around us in the moonlight. The road was dark and ahead we could see the winking indicator lights of the support cars, flickering in a long line for miles, marking out the road stretching ahead.

Knowing that night-time running has never been my strongest skill, all I could think about was making the 50-mile cut-off in time; if I didn't make it, then I would be out of the race. There were still another 84 miles after this, and I was mindful about not wanting to fall to pieces too soon by running too quickly at the start, so I tried to run neither too quickly or too slowly.

The crew fell into a cadence of stopping every 2 miles and attending to me. It took a few goes until it was as efficient as an F1 pit stop: drink bottles swapped out, food ('Eat! You must keep eating!'), a sponge down on the arms. I ate whatever they offered me: small bits of cheese, fruit, a portion of tortilla wrap, a cup of mashed potato. The crew pulled over and the car was twinkling with the fairy lights we had decorated it with, making it stand out on the dusty roadside, distinguishing it from other crew cars and giving me a visible goal. I ran towards it, neither too fast nor too slow, and a crew member was waiting for me. We repeated this, over and over on the dark desert road.

Occasionally the crew had to drive further out of sight, which I did not like. The roadside sand of the desert was sometimes too deep to drive in and out of safely (especially with a nail wedged in the tyre). Sometimes there was already another crew car in the plum spot. I tried not to worry when I could not see them, but there was a comfort knowing that they were never too far away. They took things in turn, diligent and mindful of each other. Over and over again through the race I acknowledged how lucky I was to have this group of people all rooting for me, all doing their best to get me to the finish.

There was absolutely nothing for miles: apart from the couple of places selling petrol and the Furnace Creek Visitor Centre, it was desolate, hundreds of miles of nothingness. I thought about how people travelled through here in wagon trains and cannot fathom the conditions they must have tolerated. No one was wearing an ice bandana back then.

Dawn broke and a twinge in my left knee became more persistent. My mind, which I could generally control well in races, started to drift towards the nagging pain. It wasn't awful, but at only 40 miles in, it was not going to play out well in the next 95. I breathed in the dusty warm dry air and refocused: *just keep on track, just keep the pace.*

Sunrise signalled the end of the first night and the beginning of a whole day of running in the direct piercing heat of the sun. I passed Furnace Creek and headed deeper into Death Valley. This would be the true heat of the race.

I was singing along to the music in my ears and, despite the knee, feeling good within myself. My eating had been on track and soon I would be able to have someone run with me.

••••

With every minute that passed, the sun rose a little higher and, with it, the temperature. At Mile 48 I had a pacer – Shaun – taking the first stint, 17 miles straight up a mountain. The climb was relentless. We climbed, slowly, steadily, sweat evaporating off our skin. I put on a huge pink hat with a wide brim, the sort of thing you might see on an old lady at the beach, and I loved it; it shaded my face but let me see the landscape around me.

Take it all in, Susie. Take it all in!

The desert never ceases to be beautiful to me. The colours and contours change as the sun arcs up and overhead. At its height in the middle of the day, the brightness washes out the colours. Time went by and as the afternoon set in and we passed through the mountains, more colour emerged, deeper reds and oranges, textured greys, plants with a richer shade of green. One thing remained the same: my path. It was mile after mile of road, the white line making the edge of the road stretch onwards, endlessly the same. There was seemingly no progress and no change, just the same white stripe step after step. I kept looking up and around me, ignoring the pinching knee pain and trying to be reasonable company for my crew, who took it in turns to run alongside me.

The 50-mile cut-off was marked by the sign announcing our altitude – 2000 feet – and we made it with a time buffer of one hour to spare. I was exactly where I thought I would be and was feeling energised still, which encouraged me.

After 17 miles up a mountain, mercifully the route changed to a descent, and it felt freeing to not be working to move upwards. I was with Chris Howe now and we ran down the other side, letting gravity do the work. It felt like I was flying along, spirits were high, we could see in the distance the long straight stretch of road that marked the hottest part of the course, the road that took us to Panamint Springs. It is hard to describe just how hot it was; there was a stillness to it, it felt heavy, like a feathered duvet preventing your ability to breathe properly. It was dizzying.

Debbie took over and chatted away as a fighter jet from the nearby military base swooped overhead and skirted at high speed around the surrounding mountain basin. The sound of it bounced about and was deafening and dramatic, and I felt so very in the moment, so very much part of the race of my dreams!

This is it! This is what I wanted to do so much!

Five miles later, making the next huge mountain ascent, suddenly the buoyancy of earlier deserted me and I got emotional. I was trying to hide my tears from Debbie. Perhaps it was the 71 miles in my legs, or maybe more simply the energy from the Pot Noodle (Chicken and Mushroom) had worn off. *Christ, this is hard.*

What the HELL is this climb now? Why is it so BLOODY HOT still? Will that sun ever just PISS OFF?

We headed towards a viewpoint called Father Crowley, named after a Catholic priest who worked in the vast area during the 1920s. The road, which is cut into the hot mountain rocks, is steep, and served me with another 9 miles of climbing. The feel-good miles of earlier were long gone.

My feet were starting to ache deeply and I was heading into the second night, knowing that this was new territory for me – further than I have ever run (beyond 103 miles) and during the night too when I was at my weakest.

The sun set; the moon rose.

I started drinking a recovery drink called horchata – a rice-based beverage, laced with cinnamon and mild spices. It tasted inoffensive and, more importantly, I could drink it without any gag reflex – both were a massive bonus this far in to the race.

After necking it, I started to feel like a new woman. The rollercoaster of ultrarunning was now at full pelt, and my crew could do nothing more than try to keep me on track, moving forward, and to humour me as the fatigue started to make me a little delirious.

I faded out, then came back about five times overnight. Oscillating wildly from running along and singing to falling asleep mid-stride, I was unable to summon up the energy to speak. Occasionally I asked to stop and my crew let me sit in a chair and shut my eyes for five-minute stints. I was never sure if I had slept or not: as soon as they told me I had to get up, my response was to stand up as quickly as physically possible and start moving as best I could.

The tarmac scars in the road turned into snakes and the bushes turned into dinosaurs. Faces popped out of the rocks. I pointed them out to Phil, sometimes laughing at how ridiculous it was, seeing a triceratops in Death Valley of all places! Sometimes the phantom snakes made me jump and I had to skip over them, not wanting to get bitten, which made my tired legs hurt, and then suddenly it was not funny at all. I started to moan incessantly about my feet hurting and repeatedly ask when dawn was.

Is that it? Is that the sun coming up?

Is that the sun?

How long until the sun comes up?

More horchata.

The crew were patient, calm and kind in the face of my increasingly absurd visions. They humoured my dinosaur chat and placated my neediness, despite battling their own second night of fatigue.

••••

'Look, Susie! Look!'

Phil pointed behind my head. My sides and body ached deeply as I turned to see the very beginnings of a new day reach into the night sky.

The pain in my feet was now excruciating. Each step hurt. A pain so deep it was like I could feel it in my marrowbone. It was like someone has sliced off the bottoms of my feet and I was now trying to run on the bare bones and raw flesh. And the knee twinge was still there, though at least it wasn't getting worse. *Perhaps it is the same and now my feet hurt more?*

We iced my knee, and my feet, which seemed to alleviate things only momentarily, and by then, 113 miles in, the thought of taking off a trainer made me feel queasy.

I saw Debbie step out the car and knew she had got out for one thing only – to get me moving better again.

We were heading along a long straight road that would take us up to Lone Pine, the last stop before the mammoth climb up Mount Whitney. I needed to start to pick things up, for myself, for my crew.

'Let's just run to that pole.' Debbie pointed at a pole about 30 metres away.

I knew if I started explaining to one of the toughest women I knew that I was feeling rather tired, she would probably try very hard to make me run to the pole anyway.

We ran to the pole, then she pointed out another. I mustered the energy. We ran some more, and then some more, and incredibly I started to feel good again; the fact that I was still running this far in boosted my confidence, so we kept going. It is astonishing what the human body can do if you will it on enough. Somehow, Debbie had managed, even this far in to the race, to get me moving well again and the miles started to tick off once more. We ran past the crew car and waved them on: 'Another mile, another mile!'

They passed us, arms flailing out the windows, waving and cheering. I felt good again!

YES, COME ON!

We reached Lone Pine, after 122 miles. This was a huge mental goal for me. I was exhausted and did I mention my feet hurt like fuck? Despite this, the stint of good running and the knowledge that the finish line was edging so much closer, my spirits started to soar as I made the left turn up the Portal Road. *This is it, the last push to the finish, just up to the top now.*

Despite the terrible searing pain of each step, despite the tiredness that had shut down any deep thoughts at all, despite the feeling that there was no part of my body which did not ache, I felt happy. I was actually happy! A deep enriching satisfaction, a real warmth in my chest like a power radiating from within. Whatever happened then – the car could spontaneously combust, my crew could stop caring, I could even, heaven forbid, run out of horchata – whatever happened now, I was so close that I knew at that moment that I was going to make it. I just knew and this gave me strength.

The crew car blasted music out as I passed, and Shaun and Debbie dancing unreservedly and shamelessly at the roadside put a smile on my face.

Chris was talking to me like I was five years old. 'Well done! Just some more steps, you are being so good!'

It was the exact level of communication I could deal with.

And I feel so very alive! *Badwater! I cannot believe this is actually happening!*

I felt like I was powering up this thing, ripping my way up the mountain − flying! The reality was the progress was so slow it looked to those following online like I had almost stopped. I switched on my phone for the first time in the race and immediately hundreds of notifications pinged. The first thing I saw was a series of messages from colleagues at work, who seemed to be in a wild flurry of excitement and support for me. I sent them a message. I realised how many people were invested in this last climb and it moved me. I felt almost overwhelmed by emotion. I could not look at any more messages. *Not right now, not yet, it's almost too much. I haven't crossed the line and I don't want to break the spell − for me, my crew and this race.*

The switchbacks got sharper, the mountain even steeper and finally . . . finally the desert gave way to pine trees and a snowy mountain top. The air cooled and freshened, and behind me was the desert landscape and the mountains we had climbed; the vastness of the route was now my backdrop. Less than one mile to go and I started to fight back a huge wave of emotion, of relief, of realisation, of exhaustion.

Twelve years. It had been a 12-year dream to make it to this finish line. All those races, all those training runs, all those miles run clouded my mind. This was it as far as I was concerned. *This is me at the pinnacle of my running. This is as good as it gets. It's happening. I've done it.*

••••

For god's sake, don't start crying, Susie. You don't want to look like a blubbering knob in the finish photos.

I quietly wiped away a tear and fell into step with my crew as we ran to the finish line. Everyone who attempts this race knows it is a team race and a team effort − you simply cannot make it alone. You are your team. We had done it, and with high grins of relief and pride we crossed the line hand in hand, breaking the tape together. I was just so happy.

'Ahhh, Susie! I knew you'd get here eventually.' Chris Kostman welcomed me with a cheeky wink and everyone clapped.

All I could say was: 'My feet hurt', which was possibly the hundredth time my crew had heard that.

The pain subsided. It always does. The tendons became less inflamed, the walking became more normal. The afterglow of success burned longer than the pain.

I found out about the nail in the tyre afterwards while having a beer in Lone Pine's bar, Jake's Saloon. I was grateful no one told me. It would have stressed me out the entire time. Yes, my feet hurt – I always knew they were going to – but somewhat unusually for me I had enjoyed the race all the way through. Even the phantom snakes and crying episodes. Normally it is not until afterwards that it becomes fun, Type 2 fun, the achievement much more enjoyable than the doing. This one was different. This was special, my own personal life goal. I had become the first European female and the first non-US resident to finish the Badwater Ultra Cup.

Afterwards I realised that at no point did I think I would not make it. I just did not entertain the thought; I never let it enter my head; it was not an outcome that I was prepared to let happen. That's because this was always going to be a one-time-only thing, a race that was not one to fail, and it was special, the pinnacle. Once and once only; never again.

••••

'So why do you run?'

I must admit, I get fed up of this question. How am I supposed to answer it?

It's not straightforward. It's not one single thing, it changes. Year to year, month to month, day to day.

Some days it is fun, some days it is a chore. Running is not a simple action to be done, it is many things.

You run through emotions, run to blank them, run to think about them. You can run away, run towards, run to be in the moment, run to take yourself away from life. Run to numb feelings, run to make yourself feel alive. Run to feel part of something, run to feel splendid isolation. It strips you down, builds you up, humbles you, it gives you confidence.

Running lifts you up and breaks your heart. Running expects nothing of you.

Some days I do not enjoy running, some days I am just doing it, and some days I go out and run and feel so connected and so free, able just to be myself.

Why do I run?

I run because I can.

There is one thing about running: it is ongoing, it changes with you and gives you back what you put in.

Did I say, *never again*?

Never say never.

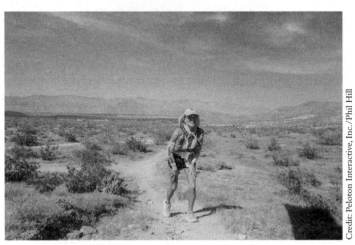

Cooking in the heat in Salton Sea.

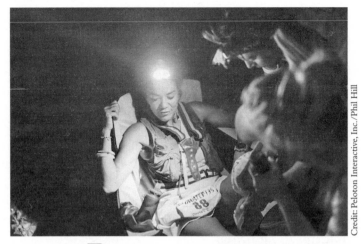

Taking a five-minute rest in the second night of no sleep.

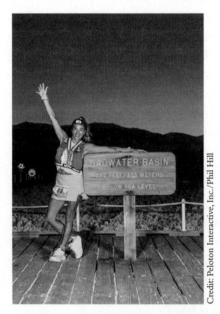

The hardest race of them all.

ACKNOWLEDGEMENTS

There are so many people to thank for this book and for fear of missing anyone out – the other day the menopause made me forget the name of a tin opener, while looking at a tin opener – I will keep it general.

Firstly, a big shout-out to all race directors and volunteers for putting events on. Without you taking the care, time and energy, thousands of people would not get to challenge themselves or have the opportunity to feel what it is like to stand at a start line or experience the magic of the running community. An extra special shout-out to race directors of the more extreme races in far-flung places, and those whose events I have not covered in this book, from local parkruns to multistage ultramarathons; so many more than I have described.

To all who have run with me in any capacity – during races, in my Peloton classes and in real life. You have no idea how much you keep me going and how you have helped me lace up my trainers on the tough days when running sucks. Suffice to say, if you are named in this book, then I give you a huge thanks for being part of the journey. There are so many more run friends who are special to me and did not make it in; it's not that you are not special, you just need to actually agree when I ask you to run an ultramarathon with me.

My family, who did not think running was an actual job and who have supported me in these endeavours, which can seem like a strange and baffling way to spend a weekend. At no point did any of you tell me I could not do these things and that I should worry about my knees. Thank you for that.

For everyone at Peloton for taking a chance on a me, not letting a simple thing like my age even be a consideration when hiring me as an instructor, and for providing me with the most rewarding, inspiring and enabling environment to work in. Thank you for actively encouraging me to run my heart out.

Huge thanks to Bloomsbury for this opportunity to write. I know I am not the fastest or, in all honesty, the best, but you have all been so supportive and reassuring, and it is with gratitude I am finally able to say thank you. It was an anxious process for me, and you made it feel so much easier and encouraged me just at the right moments.

And lastly, to those I live with, who just know that running is as much a part of my daily routine as waking up, going to sleep, and leaving muddy socks and trainers all over the place. For never questioning and only supporting despite the endless hours I was out running and not being at home, thank you from the bottom of my heart!

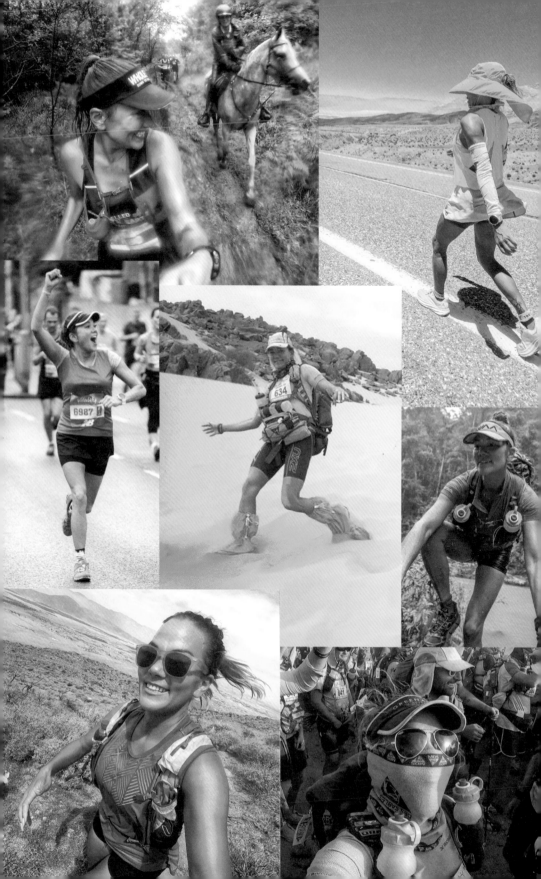